1st EDITION

Perspectives on Diseases and Disorders

Diabetes

Tom and Gena Metcalf
Book Editors

GREENHAVEN PRESS
A part of Gale, Cengage Learning

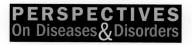

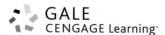

Detroit • New York • San Francisco • New Haven, Conn • Waterville, Maine • London

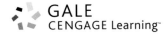

© 2008 Gale, a part of Cengage Learning

For more information, contact:
Greenhaven Books
27500 Drake Rd.
Farmington Hills, MI 48331-3535
Or you can visit our Internet site at gale.cengage.com

96 94 OCT 2 4 2008

LIBRARY OF CONGRESS CATALOGING-IN-PUBLICATION DATA

ISBN-13: 978-0-7377-3871-1

Libary of Congress Control Number: 2007940451

ISBN-10: 0-7377-3871-5

Printed in the United States of America
3 4 5 6 7 12 11 10 09 08

CONTENTS

CHAPTER 3   Personal Perspectives on Diabetes

INTRODUCTION

Over 20 million Americans, or 7 percent of the U.S. population, live with diabetes, and the number is growing. Most of the cases of diabetes—as many as 90 percent—are type 2. The number of patients diagnosed with this form of diabetes has doubled in the last decade, and that number is estimated to double again by the year 2025. Type 2 diabetes is a social and health-care system time bomb, even though the disease is avoidable and preventable in most cases.

Unlike type 1 diabetes, which appears suddenly, usually in children and young adults, type 2 diabetes takes years to develop. Type 2 is also known as adult-onset diabetes because most of the people who suffer from it are over forty-five. However, a minority of sedentary and overweight children, some as young as five, are diagnosed with type 2 diabetes.

Unlike type 1, this form of diabetes develops slowly, so slowly in fact that many people have it, do not know it, and discover it quite by accident during a doctor's visit for some other ailment. In addition, as many as 50 million people have a condition known as prediabetes, a state where symptoms are beginning to appear but the full-blown disease has not yet become apparent.

While type 1 diabetes occurs because the pancreas stops producing insulin, the conditions are different for type 2. Two factors are involved. The first is the reduction of insulin production by the pancreas. Doctors offer no specific reason for this. In some cases it is disease or age related, but in other instances the reason is unidentifiable. The second factor is insulin resistance. The body's cells become less sensitive to insulin and so the hormone's ability to signal cells to accept glucose for energy is impaired. These changes occur very slowly, but the danger for patients with this condition is significant. Prediabetes is linked to cardiovascular disease and the increased risk of strokes and heart attacks.

Genetics is a risk factor for type 2 diabetes but does not provide a complete explanation. The Pima Indians live in Arizona and adjacent to Mexico. Those who live in Mexico eat a traditional high-fiber diet and are physically active. The Pimas in Arizona eat food that is typically American—high in fat and calories. The Pimas on both sides of the border are genetically the same. Yet the incidence of type 2 diabetes is much higher on the American side than it is on the Mexican side.

The trend toward a more sedentary lifestyle is also a suspected risk factor. One hundred years ago, most of the

Improving awareness can help many people prevent the onset of type 2 diabetes. (**AP Images.**)

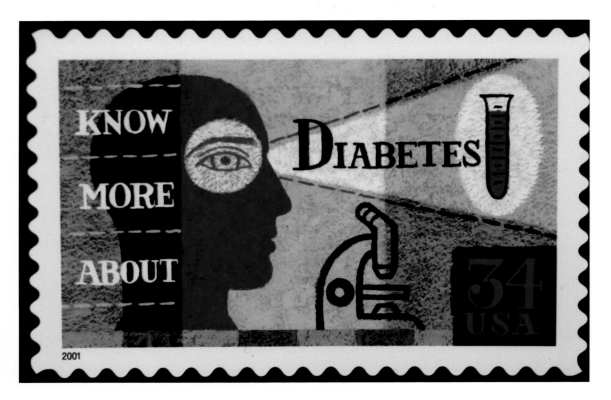

population lived on farms and engaged in physical labor. Today, most adults spend their workdays sitting, frequently in front of computers. Time away from work offers little physical activity. Researchers at the University of California at Berkeley found that Americans are nine times more likely to watch television or movies than engage in sports and physical activities.

Patterns of inactivity begin at an early age. A recent study at Johns Hopkins School of Medicine revealed that one-fifth of the children in the study engaged in two or fewer vigorous activities a week—much less than deemed healthy. Furthermore, they found that 26 percent of U.S. children spend four or more hours a day watching television.

Children's weight, the researchers concluded, was directly proportional to the amount of time they spent watching television. With inactivity and obesity comes an increased risk of type 2 diabetes.

Television watching adversely affects children with type 1 diabetes, too. A study conducted at the University of Oslo, Norway, found that excessive television watching is associated with poor blood sugar control. The rapid rise in the incidence of diabetes has led many in the medical community to call it a crisis. While many more cases of diabetes are diagnosed, some of the increase may be due to better diagnostic methods. The medical community has changed the blood sugar standard for determining diabetes twice in recent years—once in 1997 and again in 2003. Changing the standards for diabetes naturally identified more people at risk of developing the disease.

While new treatments make most type 2 diabetes cases manageable, the disease largely remains preventable through improved lifestyle and diet. It is a sobering thought that as people are able to work less and enjoy life more, they are developing habits that ultimately may take years off their lives.

CHAPTER 1

Understanding Diabetes

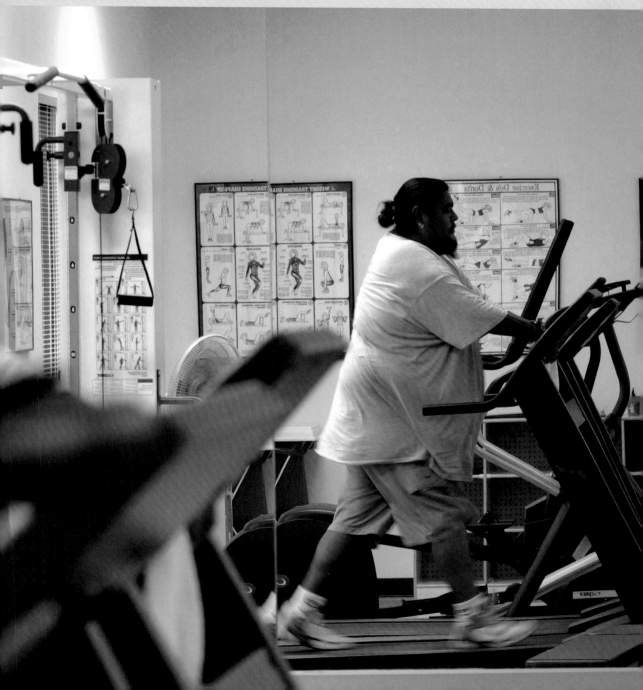

The Scope of the Problem

Altha Roberts Edgren and Teresa G. Odle

Seventeen million Americans have diabetes and only half of them know it, according to this selection by Altha Roberts Edgren and Teresa G. Odle. The authors explain that the disease is caused by the pancreas failing to create enough insulin for the body to process glucose in the bloodstream. Edgren and Odle thus describe the three kinds of diabetes: Type 1 begins most frequently in childhood. Type 2, less severe, develops in adults, often in people who are overweight and do not exercise. Gestational diabetes affects pregnant women and usually vanishes after delivery. The authors highlight the causes and symptoms of diabetes as well as the treatment and prognosis. Edgren and Odle are medical writers.

D iabetes mellitus is a condition in which the pancreas no longer produces enough insulin or cells stop responding to the insulin that is produced,

Photo on previous page. Many doctors see a strong link between the rise in obesity among Americans and an increase in type 2 diabetes. (**AP Images.**)

SOURCE: Altha Roberts Edgren and Teresa G. Odle. From "Diabetes Mellitus," in *The Gale Encyclopedia of Medicine.* Third Edition. Edited by Jacqueline L. Longe. Thomson Gale, 2006. Reproduced by permission of Thomson Gale.

so that glucose in the blood cannot be absorbed into the cells of the body. Symptoms include frequent urination, lethargy, excessive thirst, and hunger. The treatment includes changes in diet, oral medications, and in some cases, daily injections of insulin.

Diabetes mellitus is a chronic disease that causes serious health complications including renal (kidney) failure, heart disease, stroke, and blindness. Approximately 17 million Americans have diabetes. Unfortunately, as many as one-half are unaware they have it.

Insulin Shortage Upsets Normal Metabolism

Every cell in the human body needs energy in order to function. The body's primary energy source is glucose, a simple sugar resulting from the digestion of foods containing carbohydrates (sugars and starches). Glucose from the digested food circulates in the blood as a ready energy source for any cells that need it. Insulin is a hormone or chemical produced by cells in the pancreas, an organ located behind the stomach. Insulin bonds to a receptor site on the outside of a cell and acts like a key to open a doorway into the cell through which glucose can enter. Some of the glucose can be converted to concentrated energy sources like glycogen or fatty acids and saved for later use. When there is not enough insulin produced or when the doorway no longer recognizes the insulin key, glucose stays in the blood rather [than] entering the cells.

The body will attempt to dilute the high level of glucose in the blood, a condition called hyperglycemia, by drawing water out of the cells and into the bloodstream in an effort to dilute the sugar and excrete it in the urine. It is not unusual for people with undiagnosed diabetes to be constantly thirsty, drink large quantities of water, and urinate frequently as their bodies try to get rid of the extra glucose. This creates high levels of glucose in the urine.

At the same time that the body is trying to get rid of glucose from the blood, the cells are starving for glucose and sending signals to the body to eat more food, thus making patients extremely hungry. To provide energy for the starving cells, the body also tries to convert fats and proteins to glucose. The breakdown of fats and proteins for energy causes acid compounds called ketones to form in the blood. Ketones also will be excreted in the urine. As ketones build up in the blood, a condition called ketoacidosis can occur. This condition can be life threatening if left untreated, leading to coma and death.

Diabetes Strikes at All Ages

Type 1 diabetes, sometimes called juvenile diabetes, begins most commonly in childhood or adolescence. In this form of diabetes, the body produces little or no insulin.

Two diabetic children have their blood sugar levels tested before lunch. (**AP Images.**)

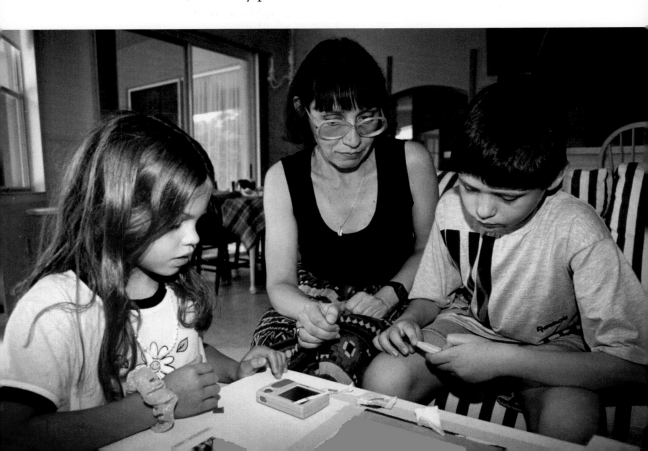

It is characterized by a sudden onset and occurs more frequently in populations descended from Northern European countries (Finland, Scotland, Scandinavia) than in those from Southern European countries, the Middle East, or Asia. In the United States, approximately three people in 1,000 develop Type 1 diabetes. This form also is called insulin-dependent diabetes because people who develop this type need to have daily injections of insulin. . . .

The more common form of diabetes, Type 2, occurs in approximately 3–5% of Americans under 50 years of age, and increases to 10–15% in those over 50. More than 90% of the diabetics in the United States are Type 2 diabetics. Sometimes called age-onset or adult-onset diabetes, this form of diabetes occurs most often in people who are overweight and who do not exercise. It is also more common in people of Native American, Hispanic, and African-American descent. People who have migrated to Western cultures from East India, Japan, and Australian Aboriginal cultures also are more likely to develop Type 2 diabetes than those who remain in their original countries.

Type 2 is considered a milder form of diabetes because of its slow onset (sometimes developing over the course of several years) and because it usually can be controlled with diet and oral medication. The consequences of uncontrolled and untreated Type 2 diabetes, however, are just as serious as those for Type 1. This form is also called noninsulin-dependent diabetes, a term that is somewhat misleading. Many people with Type 2 diabetes can control the condition with diet and oral medications, however, insulin injections are sometimes necessary if treatment with diet and oral medication is not working.

Another form of diabetes called gestational diabetes can develop during pregnancy and generally resolves after the baby is delivered. This diabetic condition devel-

FAST FACT

In 2005 an estimated 20.8 million people in the United States had diabetes. Of all the cases, 14.6 million were diagnosed and 6.2 million were undiagnosed.

ops during the second or third trimester of pregnancy in about 2% of pregnancies. . . .

Diabetes also can develop as a result of pancreatic disease, alcoholism, malnutrition, or other severe illnesses that stress the body.

The Causes of Diabetes Are Murky

The causes of diabetes mellitus are unclear; however, there seem to be both hereditary (genetic factors passed on in families) and environmental factors involved. Research has shown that some people who develop diabetes have common genetic markers. In Type 1 diabetes, the immune system, the body's defense system against infection, is believed to be triggered by a virus or another microorganism that destroys cells in the pancreas that produce insulin. In Type 2 diabetes, age, obesity, and family history of diabetes play a role.

In Type 2 diabetes, the pancreas may produce enough insulin; however, cells have become resistant to the insulin produced and it may not work as effectively. Symptoms of Type 2 diabetes can begin so gradually that a person may not know that he or she has it. Early signs are lethargy, extreme thirst, and frequent urination. Other symptoms may include sudden weight loss, slow wound healing, urinary tract infections, gum disease, or blurred vision. It is not unusual for Type 2 diabetes to be detected while a patient is seeing a doctor about another health concern that is actually being caused by the yet undiagnosed diabetes.

Individuals who are at high risk of developing Type 2 diabetes mellitus include people who:

- are obese (more than 20% above their ideal body weight)
- have a relative with diabetes mellitus
- belong to a high-risk ethnic population (African-American, Native American, Hispanic, or Native Hawaiian)

Estimated Total Prevalence of Diabetes

This graph shows the estimated percentage of people in the United States with diabetes, diagnosed and undiagnosed, as of 2002.

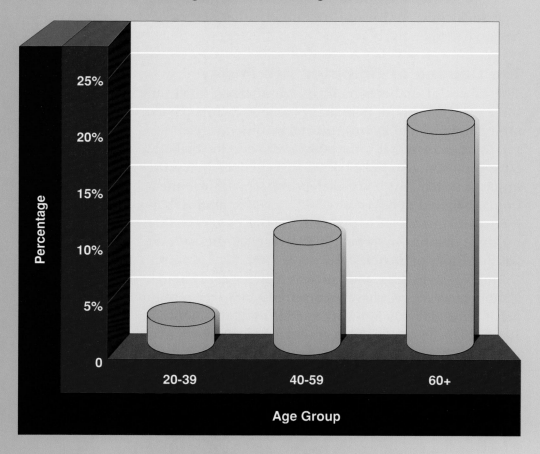

Source: 1999–2002 National Health and Nutrition Examination Survey.

- have been diagnosed with gestational diabetes or have delivered a baby weighing more than 9 lbs (4 kg)
- have high blood pressure (140/90 mmHg or above)
- have a high density lipoprotein cholesterol level less than or equal to 35 mg/dL and/or a triglyceride level greater than or equal to 250 mg/dL

PERSPECTIVES ON DISEASES AND DISORDERS

• have had impaired glucose tolerance or impaired fasting glucose on previous testing. . . .

Symptoms and Diagnosis

Symptoms of diabetes can develop suddenly (over days or weeks) in previously healthy children or adolescents, or can develop gradually (over several years) in overweight adults over the age of 40. The classic symptoms include feeling tired and sick, frequent urination, excessive thirst, excessive hunger, and weight loss.

Ketoacidosis, a condition due to starvation or uncontrolled diabetes, is common in Type 1 diabetes. Ketones are acid compounds that form in the blood when the body breaks down fats and proteins. Symptoms include abdominal pain, vomiting, rapid breathing, extreme lethargy, and drowsiness. Patients with ketoacidosis will also have a sweet breath odor. Left untreated, this condition can lead to coma and death.

With Type 2 diabetes, the condition may not become evident until the patient presents for medical treatment for some other condition. A patient may have heart disease, chronic infections of the gums and urinary tract, blurred vision, numbness in the feet and legs, or slow-healing wounds. Women may experience genital itching.

Diabetes is suspected based on symptoms. Urine tests and blood tests can be used to confirm a diagnosis of diabetes based on the amount of glucose found. Urine can also detect ketones and protein in the urine that may help diagnose diabetes and assess how well the kidneys are functioning. These tests also can be used to monitor the disease once the patient is on a standardized diet, oral medications, or insulin. . . .

Diabetes Can Have Severe Consequences

There is currently no cure for diabetes. The condition, however, can be managed so that patients can live a relatively normal life. Treatment of diabetes focuses on two goals: keeping blood glucose within normal range and preventing the development of long-term complications. Careful monitoring of diet, exercise, and blood glucose levels are as important as the use of insulin or oral medications in preventing complications of diabetes. In 2003, the American Diabetes Association updated its Standards of Care for the management of diabetes. These standards help managed health care providers in the most recent recommendations for diagnosis and treatment of the disease. . . .

Uncontrolled diabetes is a leading cause of blindness, end-stage renal disease, and limb amputations. It also doubles the risks of heart disease and increases the risk of stroke. Eye problems including cataracts, glaucoma, and diabetic retinopathy also are more common in diabetics.

Diabetic peripheral neuropathy is a condition where nerve endings, particularly in the legs and feet, become less sensitive. Diabetic foot ulcers are a particular problem since the patient does not feel the pain of a blister, callus, or other minor injury. Poor blood circulation in the legs and feet contribute to delayed wound healing. The inability to sense pain along with the complications of delayed wound healing can result in minor injuries, blisters, or calluses becoming infected and difficult to treat. In cases of severe infection, the infected tissue begins to break down and rot away. The most serious consequence of this condition is the need for amputation of toes, feet, or legs due to severe infection.

New Treatments for Diabetes

Terri D'Arrigo

Terri D'Arrigo is an associate editor of *Diabetes Forecast* magazine, published by the American Diabetic Association. In this viewpoint D'Arrigo examines state-of-the-art treatments for diabetes. Most of these developments are with groundbreaking medications. She gives an overview of several drugs that help to promote insulin production. D'Arrigo also reports on continuous glucose monitoring systems that are becoming available. The common problem with all these treatments is their cost. Generally they are expensive, and many are not covered by insurance plans.

Diabetes management is constantly evolving. Every year, new drugs come onto the market, many of which are updated versions of existing products. But recent years have seen the birth of several classes of drugs that work in new and different ways. There are

SOURCE: Terri D'Arrigo, "Trailblazers: Recent Years Have Seen the Addition of Several New Classes of Diabetes Drugs . . . ," *Diabetes Forecast*, vol. 60, March 2007, p. 32–4. Copyright © 2007 American Diabetes Association. Reproduced by permission.

pros and cons to each, and because they're all still relatively new, the jury is out on their long-term effects. That said, here's the inside scoop from some health care professionals who have experience prescribing them.

Inhalable Insulin Offers Greater Freedom

Exubera has made the biggest splash in publicity, and with good reason: It's the first inhalable insulin. It comes in measured packets of powder that you place into an inhaler. Exubera is a rapid-acting insulin and should be taken no more than 10 minutes before a meal, and it may be used to treat both type 1 and type 2 diabetes. If your diabetes care plan includes the use of injected basal insulin, you would continue using that as well.

The freedom to take fewer shots comes with a price, however, says Irl B. Hirsch, MD, professor of medicine at the University of Washington Medical Center–Roosevelt in Seattle. "Most insurance doesn't cover it yet," he says. "Once it's on the market a while, maybe insurers will be a little more kind."

Several diabetes drugs require follow-up tests—the thiazolidinedione (TZD or "glitazone") class of type 2 drugs requires liver tests and metformin requires creatinine tests—but the lung tests required for Exubera might not always be convenient, says Hirsch. If your doctor doesn't have access to the right equipment, he or she may have to refer you to another doctor or clinic.

So far, Exubera has not made the impact many experts thought it might. "If it had arrived 4 or 5 years ago, it might have a bigger place in practice than it does now," says Matthew C. Riddle, MD, professor of medicine and head of the section of diabetes in the division of endocrinology at the Oregon Health and Science University in Portland. "The alternatives to its use have been proved over time—more people are using insulin pens and drugs like Byetta. I don't think it will replace injected insulin dramatically. It's not bad, however. It just means we have more options."

Hormone Management Drugs

DPP-4 inhibitors, the newest class of type 2 drugs, help maintain levels of the gut hormone GLP- 1. When you eat, your small intestines secrete GLP-1, which then promotes insulin production by the pancreas. DPP-4 breaks down GLP-1. In people without diabetes, that's good because it prevents the overproduction of insulin. But people with diabetes often have a deficiency of GLP-1, so turning DPP-4 off will allow the GLP-1 they do have to work longer in promoting insulin secretion.

While a variety of new treatments for diabetes are being developed, many are prohibitively expensive.
(**AP Images.**)

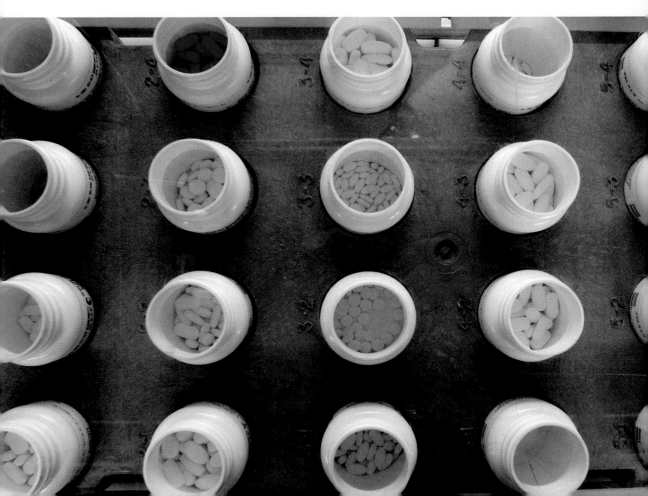

Januvia (sitagliptin) is the first DPP-4 inhibitor to be approved by the U.S. Food and Drug Administration. Several other DPP-4 inhibitors are likely to come to the market within the next few years.

DPP-4 inhibitors are being marketed as competition for sulfonylureas, but the burden of proof is on the companies that make this new class, says Riddle. Although DPP-4 inhibitors don't cause low blood glucose or weight gain—older sulfonylureas may—whether they stack up against newer sulfonylureas remains to be seen, he says. "Overall, DPP-4 inhibitors appear not to be any more powerful, and perhaps less so than metformin and certain sulfonylureas."

Again, cost rears its ugly head. "They're extremely expensive, roughly 4 or 5 dollars a day," says Hirsch. "They will fall into [the highest co-pay] for many insurance plans. With sulfonylureas [in the lowest co-pay] or generic, I don't think the average person is going to be willing to pay more."

Yet DPP-4 inhibitors offer hope: Some animal studies suggest they may help the insulin-producing beta cells in the pancreas survive and grow. There have not been any studies to determine if DPP-4 inhibitors might help preserve human beta cells, but the potential payoff could be big, says Stuart T. Haines, PharmD, BC-ADM, CDE, professor at the University of Maryland School of Pharmacy and clinical specialist at the Joslin Diabetes Center at the University of Maryland Medical Center in Baltimore. "It would be a huge breakthrough in how we treat diabetes," he says. "We could then prescribe them early in the course of the disease to counteract the process."

New Drugs Can Be Unpredictable

Byetta (exenatide) is an injectable type 2 drug for people who take thiazolidinediones (TZDs), metformin, a sulfonylurea, or a combination of metformin and a

---

FAST FACT

Medco Health Solutions Inc. projects that by 2009, spending on medicines to treat diabetes could increase by 60-68 percent from 2006 levels.

---

sulfonylurea. It's the first in a class of drugs called incretin mimetics, and it mimics the action of GLP-1. Byetta should be taken less than an hour before the morning and evening meals.

So far, it appears that Byetta is the sleeper among new diabetes drugs—it's enough of a hit that there was a shortage of it in early 2006. "It has exceeded people's expectations," says Riddle. "It works better than a lot of people thought it would, particularly in terms of weight loss."

The average weight loss is about 10 to 15 pounds over a few years, says Hirsch, but some people have lost considerably more, up to 40 or 50 pounds.

"The trouble is you can't predict the weight loss," says Hirsch. "It's not from nausea [a known temporary side effect]. It appears to take away the appetite."

Riddle adds that not all insurance companies cover it, and preauthorization is routine.

Confusion of Multiple Medicines

Symlin (pramlintide acetate) is an injectable synthetic analog of the human hormone amylin and is approved for people with type 1 or type 2 who use insulin. It slows the release of food from the stomach into the intestines, slows the production of glucose by the liver, and helps control appetite. (Byetta has these same effects.) Symlin should be taken just before a meal.

On the plus side, Symlin may lower the amount of insulin you have to take and can help promote weight loss. The caveat is that if you take insulin by injection, you're adding more shots to your care regimen, and that can wear on you, says Haines. "Basically, now you're giving multiple, multiple daily injections," he says.

He adds that because Symlin doesn't come in a prefilled syringe and the dosing doesn't correspond directly to the units on an insulin syringe, there's a potential for confusion among doctors, pharmacists, and people who use the drug alike.

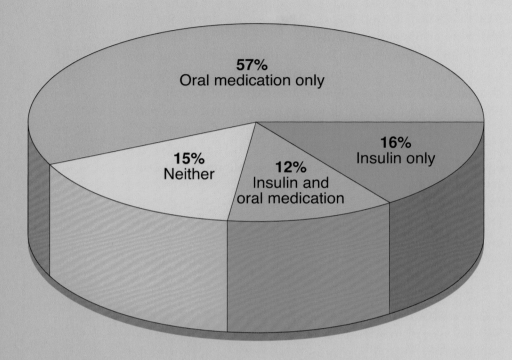

Medication of Adults with Diabetes in the United States 2001–2003

57%
Oral medication only

15%
Neither

12%
Insulin and oral medication

16%
Insulin only

Source: 2001–2003 National Health Interview Survey.

"Still, it does have a place," says Haines. "It seems to do a good job of smoothing out after-meal high blood glucose."

All in all, these new classes of drugs provide new options, says Riddle. "But don't forget that existing options are pretty good. We need proof that the newer options are better before we go overboard," he says.

The good news is that once the first drug in a class gains some momentum, there's often a flurry of "me too" drugs, says Haines, and that can work to your advantage. "There will most likely be several drugs in each class, with subtle differences between them such as how many times a day you take them or the price. Once one company makes a drug, the others often try to make it better. As more drugs compete, the price will go down as managed care and insurance companies take their business to the companies with the most affordable drugs."

If history repeats itself, these new classes of drugs are clearing the path for further evolution in diabetes treatment.

New Monitors Promise Better Control

All that's new in diabetes management is not pharmaceutical. Continuous glucose monitoring has arrived, albeit in a somewhat limited fashion as manufacturers make their products available one city at a time.

The components of each system vary, but all include a sensor that is inserted under the skin through a probe. The sensor measures glucose in interstitial fluid (fluid around cells) and delivers readings every few minutes. All continuous glucose monitoring systems have alarms to alert you to high or low blood glucose, although experts agree that you should do a fingerstick test before treating either condition.

"These systems can benefit people with diabetes who are highly motivated to take tight control of their blood glucose or who have trouble with lows," says . . . Hirsch. . . . "The big issue is cost: Insurance companies aren't paying for them."

As with drugs, coverage may increase as these systems become more common and less expensive.

The Search for a Cure for Type 1 Diabetes

Juvenile Diabetes Research Foundation

The Juvenile Diabetes Research Foundation (JDRF) was founded in 1970 by parents of children with diabetes. It has raised over $1 billion for research into the disease. The JDRF notes in the following viewpoint that while a cure for the disease has eluded researchers, treatment and quality of life have improved for people who have the disease. The JDRF has two functions: to eradicate the disease and to reduce the life-threatening aspects of it. It states that glucose control is the central issue in both.

Medical research to discover cures for diabetes and its complications, while not yet resulting in widespread treatments to reverse the disease, has already had a positive impact on the quality of life for people with type 1 diabetes. On the path toward therapeutic cures, research has refocused medical care on

SOURCE: Originally appeared in *Countdown*, Winter 2007, a publication of Juvenile Diabetes Research Foundation International, www.jdrf.org. Reproduced by permission.

how diabetes is managed, resulting in a lower risk of complications and longer life expectancy, particularly for those diagnosed today. At the same time, the development of a range of drugs, treatments, and diagnostic tools has slowed the impact of some complications for people with type 1.

The research leading to improvements in quality of life—some measured, others more significant—has taken many forms. Some were large trials conducted by the NIH and other government science agencies. Others involved scientific investigation by companies that manufacture insulin, monitors, and insulin-delivery tools.

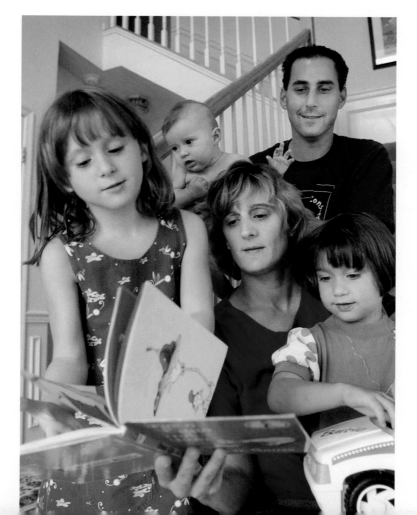

Five-year-old Jamie Langbein, left, reads with her family. Diagnosed with type 1 diabetes at the age of two, Jamie must have her fingertips pricked ten times daily to check her blood sugar levels. (**AP Images.**)

And some were traditional, academic research projects looking at the causes and treatment of diabetes, as well as complications including heart disease and kidney disease. Despite not yet achieving a cure, research has made diabetes a different disease today than it was 50, 25, or even 10 years ago. And many recent scientific advances have made life with diabetes a somewhat less daunting task than it was for previous generations. Standards of care, drugs, devices, and treatments are changing how—and how long—people with type 1 live.

The Search for a Cure

JDRF's primary focus is cure: eliminating type 1 diabetes in the way that smallpox and polio have been eradicated from most of the earth. But the commitment to a cure has always focused not just on the long-term and generational needs of people with type 1 diabetes, but also on improving their lives today by reducing the life-threatening aspects of this disease. JDRF's cure therapeutics approach to science incorporates short-term outcomes into its longer-term vision of a cure.

Diabetes research has taken two parallel paths: The first is the effort to cure the disease, prevent its occurrence and recurrence, and stop or reverse its long-term complications. Concurrently, researchers have been examining how life with diabetes is managed, focusing on ways to improve the methodology, drugs, and technology of diabetes care. The two paths are not mutually exclusive. Discoveries in one area often lead to improved treatments in another, and results achieved in diabetes treatment have reinforced or challenged ideas under development by academic researchers. The benefits aren't limited to diabetes: As scientists learn more about the molecular mechanisms of a range

FAST FACT

Between twelve thousand and twenty-four thousand cases of blindness each year are caused by diabetic retinopathy. Diabetes is the primary cause of blindness for people twenty to seventy-four years old.

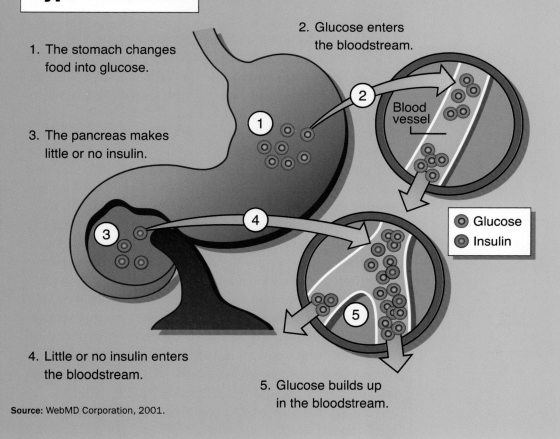

Type 1 Diabetes

1. The stomach changes food into glucose.

2. Glucose enters the bloodstream.

3. The pancreas makes little or no insulin.

Blood vessel

4. Little or no insulin enters the bloodstream.

5. Glucose builds up in the bloodstream.

◎ Glucose
◎ Insulin

Source: WebMD Corporation, 2001.

of diseases, drugs created to treat different illnesses have been discovered to have beneficial effects when used as treatments for diabetic complications.

Reducing Life-Threatening Complications

The key point of interconnection between short- and long-term research in type 1 diabetes is glucose control. Research in the pathology of diabetes and its various complications has consistently gravitated toward glucose control as the key element in the progression of heart disease, hypoglycemia, retinopathy, kidney disease, and neuropathy.

Studying Autoimmune Processes

In the 1970s, scientists first discovered that type 1 diabetes is an autoimmune disease. That discovery set in motion the careful advance through discovery science in an effort to unlock the mechanisms of the autoimmune process, and then figure out a way to interrupt it and prevent the onset of diabetes.

What followed in the case of autoimmunity research—and the same model would pertain for many areas of type 1 diabetes science—were years of lab testing, and the identification of potential therapeutics; those findings lead to proof of concept studies, and animal trials, followed by safety and efficacy-measuring tests; then come small scale human trials, and if results are encouraging at that stage, are followed by confirming studies with larger groups. As the project progresses, the research will likely have attracted the interest of pharmaceutical companies, who naturally are interested in having a stake in potential benefits of releasing a new treatment onto the market. This description captures the current state on anti-CD3 research being conducted at JDRF centers.

As JDRF-funded research becomes more development-oriented—moving from research to reality—we've highlighted some of the ways the scientific process has led to therapeutic progress.

Discrimination in the Workplace

Richmond Times-Dispatch

The following article from Virginia's *Richmond Times-Dispatch* looks at job discrimination against diabetics. It recounts the case of John Steigauf, a UPS mechanic who was fired from his job because he had diabetes. Steigauf is one of many, according to the article, who are facing job pressures because of the disease. People with diabetes are legally barred from some occupations such as military, police, commercial pilot, and truck driver. The article states that some hide their diabetes from employers, fearing discrimination. Complaints are likely to increase, the article says, because the number of people with diabetes is rising. Resolution of such complaints is difficult, according to the article, because prejudice and discrimination are hard to prove.

John Steigauf spent more than a decade fiddling with the innards of those huge United Parcel Service trucks. One icy day two years ago, the company put

SOURCE: "Diabetes Is Made a Work Issue," *Richmond Times-Dispatch*, January 6, 2007, p. B11. Copyright © Richmond Newspapers, Incorporated, January 6, 2007. Reproduced by permission.

him on leave from his mechanic's job. A supervisor escorted him off the premises. His work was good. He hadn't socked the boss or embezzled money. It had to do with what was inside him: diabetes.

UPS called it a safety issue: Steigauf's blood sugar might suddenly plummet while he tested a truck, causing him to hit someone. Steigauf considered it discrimination, a taint that diabetes can carry. "I was regarded as a damaged piece of meat," he said. "It was like, 'You're one of those, and we can't have one of those.'"

Workplace Discrimination Complaints

With 21 million American diabetics, disputes like this have increasingly rippled through the workplace. Since 1999, the American Diabetes Association has received calls from 35 Virginians regarding workplace discrimination issues, spokeswoman Diane Tuncer said. More than two-thirds of those calls were received since January 2004. Those are just the calls that Tuncer said warranted further guidance or legal assistance for the individuals. It does not include all the calls from Virginia that the group might have received to its national hot line. Diabetics contend they are being blocked by their employers from the near-normal lives their doctors say are possible. But the companies say they are struggling, too, with confusion about whether diabetes is a legitimate disability and with concern about whether it is overly expensive, hazardous and disruptive to accommodate the illness.

The debate will probably intensify. The number of diabetics in America swelled by 80 percent in the past decade. Experts say the disease is on its way to becoming a fact of life in the nation's labor force, raising all sorts of issues for workers and managers.

Many Workers Fear Reprisals

Wary of bad outcomes, many diabetics conceal their illness on the job. Brian T. McMahon, a professor at Vir-

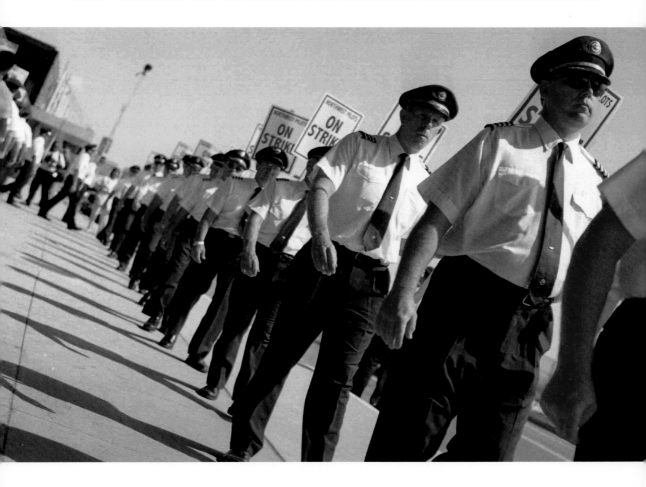

ginia Commonwealth University who studies workplace discrimination, said: "You get to the question of whether or not to disclose you have diabetes. Most people opt not to, for they fear: 'Am I inviting more trouble?'" Doctors say that with improved medications and methods of self-testing blood sugar, most diabetics can do almost any job if they properly manage their illness. Nonetheless, the risk of plunging blood sugars has long fueled a reluctance to employ diabetics in jobs such as those of truck driver or police officer, if they are on insulin.

Federal law bars diabetics from joining the armed services and prevents diabetics on insulin from becoming

People with diabetes who take insulin are legally barred from some professions, including that of commercially licensed airline pilots.
(AP Images.)

commercial pilots. However, innumerable diabetics are engaged in more mundane jobs uninvolved in matters of life and death. For these people—secretaries and factory workers and programmers—a "reasonable accommodation," like permission to eat at one's desk or to be excused

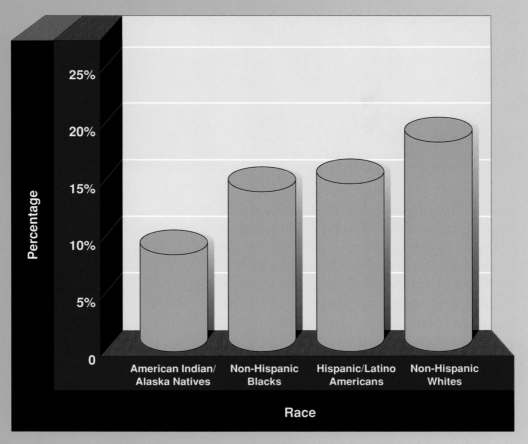

Diabetes by Race and Ethnicity

This chart shows the estimated age-adjusted total prevalence of diabetes in people aged twenty years or older, by race/ethnicity in the United States.

Source: American Diabetes Association, 2005.

from fluctuating shifts, can make the difference in whether they can function.

Complaints End Up in the Legal System

When disputes can't be resolved, the cases often land in court or before the Equal Employment Opportunity Commission. The commission, which enforces the Americans With Disabilities Act of 1990, says diabetes-related complaints have been on the rise, one of the few conditions generally showing an increase in complaints. Diabetes accounts for nearly 5 percent of the 15,000 annual cases that the EEOC gets under that act, trailing only back impairment, other orthopedic injuries and depression.

Often the courts are of scant help in bringing clarity. Judges in nearly identical cases have ruled in opposite ways, leaving diabetics bewildered and businesses unsure [of] what, if anything, they should do.

The American Diabetes Association fields about 100 calls a month about workplace tussles. Many of them revolve around accommodations, though the changes sought tend to be modest: predictable hours, a place to test blood, freedom to snack when sugars get unbalanced. However, employers prevail in a majority of cases. Many others are settled. It is hard even to get lawyers to pursue complaints, because prejudice is tricky to prove. Establishing discrimination has become harder since 1999, when the Supreme Court held that if a disability can be corrected with medicine, it is not necessarily protected. Advocates for the disabled say the ruling warped the intent of Congress.

FAST FACT

In the case of a San Antonio, Texas, man who was denied a job as a policeman because of his diabetes, the courts ruled it unlawful to disqualify a job candidate for that reason.

Stem Cell Treatment Could Reverse Type 1 Diabetes

Karen Kaplan

Karen Kaplan is a staff writer for the *Los Angeles Times*. In this article she describes a revolutionary treatment for halting and possibly reversing the onset of type 1 diabetes. Diabetes occurs, Kaplan explains, because the body's own immune system destroys the insulin-producing cells of the pancreas. In this treatment doctors extract stem cells from the patients' own bone marrow. Kaplan explains how the doctors administer chemotherapy to destroy the patients' immune systems before restoring the stem cells to them. After their immune systems recover, most of the patients are able to live without insulin. The long-term effectiveness of the treatment is unknown, according to Kaplan. While substantial risks are involved she concludes that the treatment offers hope for the future.

Researchers have demonstrated for the first time that the progression of Type 1 diabetes can be halted—and possibly reversed—by a stem-cell transplant that preserves the body's diminishing ability to make insulin, according to a study published [on April 11, 2007].

The experimental therapy eliminated the need for insulin injections for months or even years in 14 of 15 patients recently diagnosed with the disease. One subject, a 30-year-old male, hasn't taken insulin since his stem-cell transplant more than three years ago, according to the study in the *Journal of the American Medical Assn.*

The study suggests a new avenue for treating the intractable disease, in which the immune system destroys insulin-producing beta cells in the pancreas. Without insulin, patients can't metabolize sugar and run the risk of developing nerve damage, cardiovascular disease, kidney failure and blindness.

Patients with Type 1 diabetes typically compensate by monitoring their blood-sugar levels every few hours and injecting themselves with insulin as many as five times a day.

After the stem-cell treatment, "patients are absolutely medication-free—they're off insulin," said Dr. Richard Burt, chief of the Division of Immunotherapy for Autoimmune Diseases at Northwestern University's Feinberg School of Medicine in Chicago and senior author of the study.

The strategy is similar to an approach that has shown some success in treating other immune system disorders, such as rheumatoid arthritis, lupus and multiple sclerosis. "We all realize that without addressing the problem at the level of the immune system, we'll never really beat Type 1 diabetes," said Dr. Francisco Prieto, who treats diabetics in his Elk Grove, Calif., practice and wasn't involved in the study. "This is very encouraging work."

Burt and his colleagues cautioned that they didn't know whether the fix was permanent and, if it was not, how long it would last. One of the subjects was insulin-free for one year but relapsed after a respiratory viral

Gastrointestinal Tract

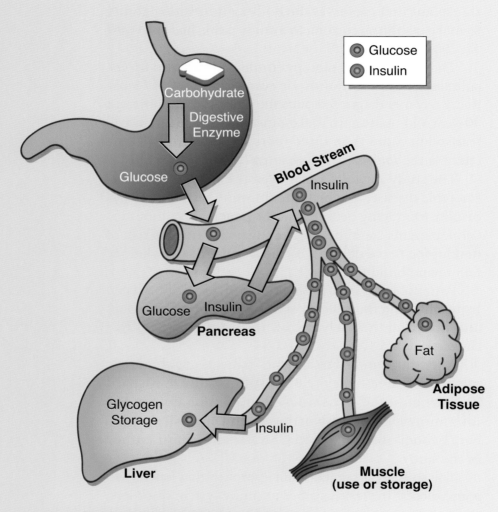

Glucose

Insulin

Carbohydrate

Digestive
Enzyme

Glucose

Blood Stream

Insulin

Glucose   Insulin

Pancreas

Fat

**Adipose
Tissue**

Glycogen
Storage

Insulin

Liver

**Muscle
(use or storage)**

Source: The Whittier Institute for Diabetes. www.whittier.org

infection, said lead author Dr. Julio Voltarelli, associate professor of medicine at Ribeirao Preto medical school at the University of Sao Paulo in Brazil.

The researchers also cautioned that the process was not without risk, because patients are vulnerable to infection during part of the therapy. Burt's research group at Northwestern has performed 170 stem-cell transplants to treat a variety of immune system disorders, and two patients have died from the treatment.

But other doctors said that even if the benefits of the therapy were temporary, the research provided valuable insight into the mechanism behind the disease. "It's a big deal," said Dr. Stephen Forman, chairman of the Division of Hematology & Hematopoietic Cell Transplantation at the City of Hope Comprehensive Cancer Center in Duarte, [California] who wasn't part of the study. "The fact that you got somebody insulin-independent, there's a clue there" for scientists in search of a cure.

Millions of Diabetics Can Benefit

The Juvenile Diabetes Research Foundation in New York estimates that as many as 3 million Americans have Type 1 diabetes, and that 30,000 to 35,000 new cases are diagnosed each year. Most of those patients will die from complications of the disease rather than from diabetes itself. The age of onset is considerably younger than for patients with Type 2 diabetes, who can still make insulin but can't use it efficiently.

> **FAST FACT**
>
> Patients with type 1 diabetes always need insulin.

The stem-cell approach mirrors the bone marrow transplants used to treat patients with certain cancers and blood diseases. Bone marrow contains hematopoietic stem cells, which are able to build all of the elements of the immune system. The idea is to wipe out the faulty immune system and replace it with a new one that functions properly.

Landmark Procedure in Brazil

In the study, 15 Brazilian patients were treated within a few months of their diagnoses, before their immune systems had the chance to eradicate all of their insulin-producing cells. The researchers hoped to preserve enough beta cells to make insulin injections unnecessary.

The study was conducted in Brazil because of Voltarelli's interest in the experiment. It was funded by the Brazilian Ministry of Health and other sources. The patients, ages 14 to 31, were treated with drugs and hormones that prompted the body to produce hematopoietic stem cells and send them from the bone marrow into the bloodstream, from which a machine then extracted them. About two weeks later, the patients checked into the hospital and received chemotherapy and other drugs to kill off their immune systems over a period of five days. Side effects for most patients included nausea, vomiting and hair loss.

After a day of rest, they were infused with their own hematopoietic stem cells, which took about eight to 12

A researcher works in a stem cell laboratory. Testing is underway to see if diabetes can be cured with stem cell infusion treatments. (AP Images.)

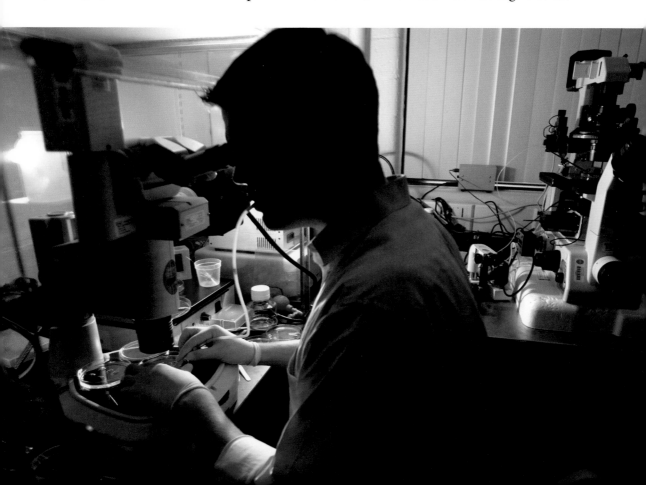

days to establish new immune systems. While the patients were without functioning immune systems, they were given antibiotics to protect them from possible infections.

The treatment had no effect on the first patient, whose disease had progressed so that his blood was dangerously acidic. He also took steroids to help him tolerate some of the drugs. After the patient's poor results, the researchers modified the study's protocol to exclude patients with his condition, called diabetic ketoacidosis, and to remove the steroids from the drug regimen.

Of the remaining 14 patients, 12 were able to stop taking insulin shortly after their transplants. Five patients have not needed insulin injections for at least 23 months, and two have been insulin-free for more than a year and a half.

One patient relapsed seven days after her transplant but gradually reduced her insulin dosage and was able to stop her injections after one year. Another patient became insulin-free 20 months after her transplant. Voltarelli said he wasn't sure why two patients had a delayed response to the transplants. "Maybe their immune systems took more time to recover and stop destroying the pancreatic" beta cells, he said.

Long-Term Results Unclear

Dr. Defu Zeng, a diabetes researcher at City of Hope, has used a similar technique to wean diabetic mice off insulin. All of the mice eventually relapsed, which leads him to suspect that the Brazilian diabetics will too. "We need to wait at least five or six years," Zeng said. "It's too early to make any conclusions."

Even if patients continue to require insulin shots, the treatment should be considered a success if it halts the destruction of beta cells, said Dr. Jay S. Skyler, associate director of the Diabetes Research Institute at the University of Miami's Miller School of Medicine, who wrote an editorial accompanying the study.

Retaining at least some insulin-producing cells makes the disease easier to control and less likely to result in severe complications, like blindness. Patients who were diagnosed with Type 1 diabetes long ago would not benefit from a stem-cell transplant because their immune systems have left nothing to preserve, he said. Some of those patients are now treated with transplants of beta cells harvested from cadavers. Scientists also are trying to use embryonic stem cells to grow beta cells for transplant.

In the long term, the treatment could potentially be combined with beta cell transplants to help patients who don't have any of their own beta cells left. If the research ultimately leads to a therapy, Prieto predicted that patients would embrace it despite the risks inherent in destroying one's immune system. "If you ask any patient with Type 1 diabetes, would they go through tremendous hardship and trials in order to be free of insulin shots, most of them would tell you yes," said Prieto, who serves on the Independent Citizens' Oversight Committee of the California Institute for Regenerative Medicine. "The risk that you could go into ketoacidosis and not survive —that's real. It happens every day."

CHAPTER 2

Controversy Surrounding Research and Treatments of Diabetes

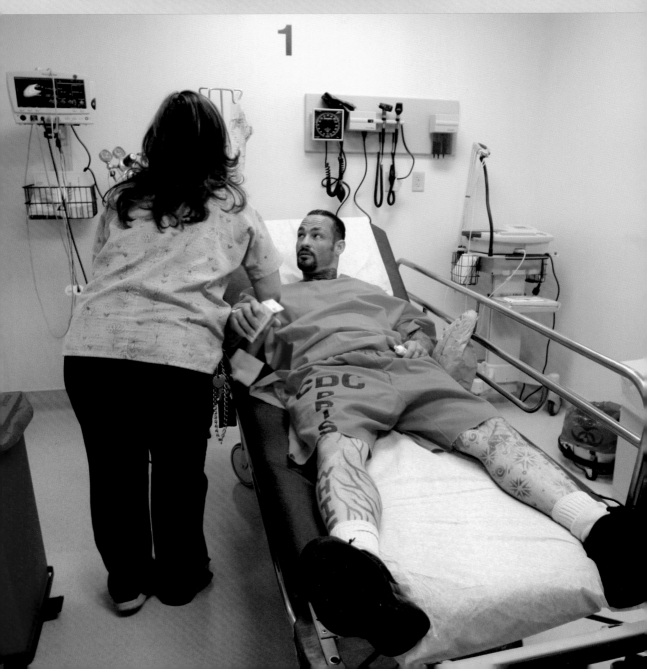

Obesity Is a Major Predictor of Type 2 Diabetes

F. Xavier Pi-Sunyer

F. Xavier Pi-Sunyer is a doctor at St. Luke's–Roosevelt Hospital Center of Columbia University. In the following article he discusses the growing trend in obesity and the close correlation between obesity and diabetes. He notes that nearly 60 percent of men and 50 percent of women in the United States are overweight or obese. Over 85 percent of type 2 diabetes patients are obese. The rate of diabetes is 2.9 percent higher in overweight people than it is in the general population. He examines the question of how obesity leads to insulin resistance. Weight loss can prevent or slow the onset of diabetes among obese patients.

Photo on previous page. An inmate receives treatment for his diabetes from a registered nurse at California's San Quentin State Prison. **(AP Images.)**

The National Health and Nutrition Examination Survey (NHANES) III, which was conducted from 1988 to 1994, showed that 59.4% of men and 50.7% of women in the United States are overweight or

SOURCE: F. Xavier Pi-Sunyer, "How Effective Are Lifestyle Changes in the Prevention of Type 2 Diabetes Mellitus?" *Nutrition Reviews,* vol. 65, March 2007, pp. 101–103, 106. Copyright © 2007 International Life Sciences Institute. Reproduced by permission.

obese. In the period from the second NHANES survey and the third, the prevalence of obesity rose from 14.5% to 22.5%. Obesity is also increasing rapidly in other parts of the world. Global obesity increased from an estimated 200 million adults in 1995 to over 300 million in 2000. Childhood obesity has also increased. During the past 30 years, childhood obesity in the United States has more than doubled. As obesity increases, it leads to an increased disease burden, leading to an increased mortality and shortened life span. Obesity brings with it not only an increased incidence of type 2 diabetes, but also of dyslipidemia, hypertension, and cardiovascular disease.

Weight as a Risk Factor

Excess weight is the most important modifiable risk factor for the development of type 2 diabetes. The incidence of diabetes rises as obesity prevalence increases. From 1990 to 1998, the prevalence of type 2 diabetes increased by 33%. There have been prospective studies describing this in Israel, Norway and Sweden. In fact, over 85% of type 2 diabetic patients are overweight or obese.

Type 2 diabetes accounts for 90% to 95% of the 16 million cases of diabetes mellitus in the United States today. The prevalence of reported diabetes is 2.9 times higher in overweight than in non-overweight persons in the NHANES data. There is a strong cross-sectional correlation between the relative weight and the prevalence of diabetes in population groups. Obesity is associated with type 2 diabetes mellitus in both women and men. Excess weight is the most important modifiable risk factor for the development of type 2 diabetes. The US National Commission on Diabetes reported that the risk of developing type 2 diabetes was about 2-fold in mildly obese, 5-fold in moderately obese, and 10-fold in severely obese people. The British Regional Heart Study, which included 7735 middle-aged men followed for 12.8 years, found that the body mass index (BMI) was the most

Arkansas governor Mike Huckabee (left) speaks to elementary school students about the need to maintain a healthy weight. Huckabee made headlines when, after being diagnosed with type 2 diabetes, he lost over one hundred pounds to better manage the disease. (**AP Images.**)

important risk factor for the development of type 2 diabetes. Men in the upper fifth of the BMI range (>27.9) had more than seven times the risk of type 2 diabetes compared with those in the lowest fifth. There is an increased risk of developing diabetes with increasing weight gain, and also an enhanced risk the higher the baseline BMI in an individual adult. Also, the longer a person remains obese, the higher the risk of his or her developing diabetes. Persons sustaining a BMI of over 30 for 10 years have twice the risk than persons who have sustained that weight for 5 years.

In both cross-sectional and longitudinal studies, fat distribution has also been found to be important in dia-

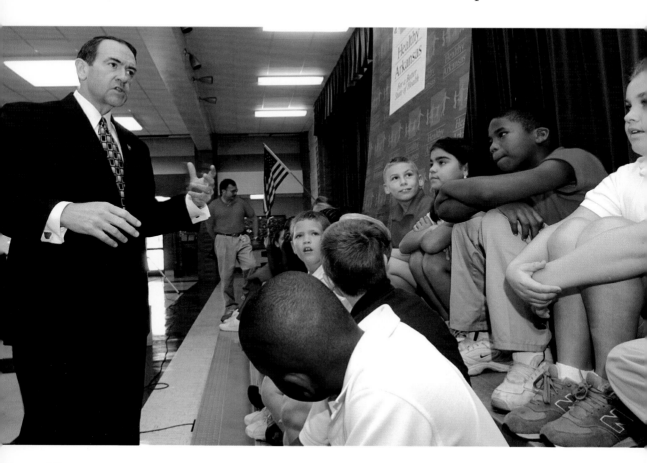

betes risk. Central or upper body fat deposition is independently associated with insulin resistance. The greater the amount of central or upper body or abdominal obesity, the greater the risk for diabetes and cardiovascular disease. Intra-abdominal or visceral obesity is strongly associated with insulin resistance, as well as with dyslipidemia, hypertension, and glucose intolerance.

In Japanese-American men, intra-abdominal fat deposition was found to be closely correlated with type 2 diabetes, while subcutaneous fat deposits in the abdomen, thorax, or thigh were not statistically significant predictors.

Lack of physical activity is another important risk factor for the development of type 2 diabetes. The British Regional Heart Study found that men who habitually engaged in moderate levels of physical activity had a substantially reduced risk of diabetes compared with physically inactive men, even after adjustment for age, BMI, and other risk factors. It is known that physical training can reduce insulin resistance and that high physical activity can lower insulin levels. Adopting a regular exercise style will also improve lipids. This is related both to an independent effect of the exercise and to a loss of fat, particularly visceral fat.

> **FAST FACT**
>
> Healthy eating, weight loss, exercise, and medication can generally control type 2 diabetes.

The Causes of Insulin Resistance

How obesity leads to insulin resistance is the subject of much controversy. Increasing weight has been associated with increasing insulin resistance. The impact of obesity is independent of genetic factors, as illustrated by a study of 23 sets of identical twins who were discordant for weight. Within twin pairs (both male and female), the obese twin had higher fasting insulin levels and showed lower insulin sensitivity than the non-obese twin. These differences were particularly evident among those with high abdominal fat distribution. . . .

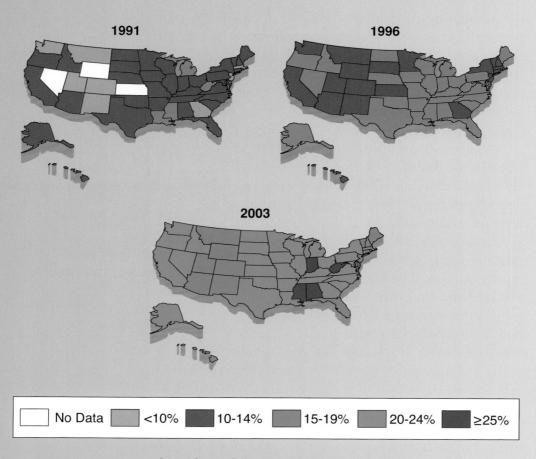

Obesity Trends Among Adults, 1991–2003

1991

1996

2003

No Data | <10% | 10-14% | 15-19% | 20-24% | ≥25%

Source: Centers for Disease Control and Prevention.

Weight Loss and Diabetes

Weight loss can prevent or delay the progression to diabetes in obese patients. In the Nurses' Health Study, women who lost more than 5 kg over a 10-year period reduced their risk of diabetes by 50% or more—a remarkable benefit for a relatively modest loss. In the Swedish Obese Subjects (SOS) study, there was a weight loss averaging 28 ± 15 kg at 2 years, and this was associated with an improvement of cardiovascular risk factors including glucose and insulin levels.

Weight loss improves insulin sensitivity, leading to lower risk factors for diabetes and cardiovascular disease. There have been a number of trials that have tested the effect of lifestyle changes on the development of diabetes in persons with IGT [impaired glucose tolerance]. These have included generally both diet and exercise to effect weight loss and improve fitness. . . .

Metabolic Syndrome and Lifestyle Changes

It has been reported that the metabolic syndrome [which includes factors such as elevated waist circumference, triglycerides, blood pressure, and glucose while fasting] increases the risk of cardiovascular disease and the risk of cardiovascular disease mortality. In the Diabetes Prevention Program [a 2002 study], 53% of the subjects had the metabolic syndrome. Of the components, an elevated waist circumference was the most common (73%) and high fasting glucose was the least common (33%). The prevalence of the metabolic syndrome between baseline and follow-up increased from 55% to 61% in the placebo group, remained unchanged in the metformin group (54% to 55%), and was reduced in the lifestyle group [those focusing on activities like weight loss and exercise] from 51% to 43%. The study showed that an intensive lifestyle intervention with weight loss and increased physical activity is more effective in reducing the onset of diabetes, but is also more effective in reducing the other components of the metabolic syndrome. This may mean that, in the long run, it is more effective in reducing the incidence of cardiovascular disease.

Obesity's Role in Type 2 Diabetes Development Is Overemphasized

Paul Campos

Paul Campos is a law professor at the University of Colorado and a nationally syndicated columnist. In this selection from his book *The Obesity Myth* Campos questions the hypothesis that obesity causes diabetes and other serious diseases. Just because obesity is correlated with the onset of diabetes does not, he argues, imply causation. Campos attributes the increase in diabetes to improved screening and reporting. He also notes that the definition of diabetes has changed, creating more cases by definition. He challenges the belief that body weight loss has a beneficial effect. In fact, he says, for many, dieting results in fluctuating weight, which is more dangerous than being obese and stable.

What about the . . . premise that, in the words of the public health establishment, being "overweight" puts a person "at risk for developing many diseases, especially heart disease, diabetes and cancer?" As we are about to see, this claim is highly misleading in two quite different ways. First, when anti-fat warriors discuss correlations between increasing body mass and various diseases, they invariably leave out the other half of the story: specifically the part that chronicles both the ambiguity of the evidence in regard to the positive correlations between fat and disease, and the many negative correlations between increasing weight and serious illness. Second, such arguments either ignore or gloss over the great difficulties that arise when one attempts to

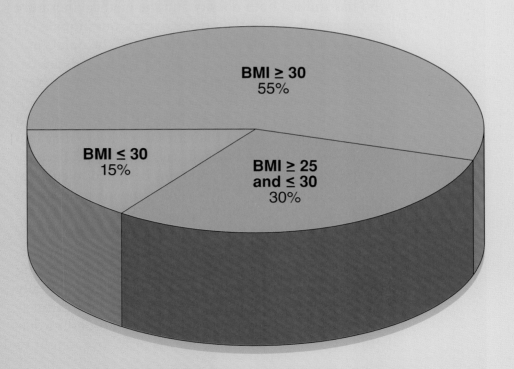

Incidence of Obesity Among People with Type 2 Diabetes

BMI ≥ 30
55%

BMI ≤ 30
15%

BMI ≥ 25
and ≤ 30
30%

Source: ObesityinAmerica.org, the Endocrine Society and the Hormone Foundation.

establish a causal, rather than a merely correlative, relationship between body mass and disease.

Let's begin by looking at [diabetes: one of] the three major diseases that are most often mentioned by those prosecuting the case against fat.

Indictments in the case against fat invariably focus on diabetes, because Type 2 diabetes is much more common among heavier-than-average people. It has become routine to claim that America is about to be overwhelmed by a diabetes epidemic, that for the first time Type 2 diabetes is being seen among children, etc., and that the solution to this crisis is to make fat people thin. The facts, however, are considerably more complicated than these claims acknowledge. Paul Ernsberger, a professor at the Case Western Reserve University School of Medicine who has studied both obesity and the medical literature regarding it for more than twenty years, questions every aspect of the conventional story. "Actually," he points out, "there is no hard data that says blood sugar levels are rising. Instead, there are many reports of telephone surveys where people are asked if they have diabetes.

Diabetes used to be tremendously under-diagnosed —less than one-third of diabetics were aware they had the disease." This has changed, says Ernsberger, because of aggressive educational programs designed to encourage more testing, and mass screenings of millions of Americans for the disease. "Also," he notes, "the definition of diabetes was changed from a fasting blood sugar of 140 to a blood sugar of 126. Thus, millions of Americans became diabetic overnight. We are also an aging population, and diabetes incidence rises exponentially after age fifty. There is also considerable confusion— many doctors are telling people they are 'borderline diabetic,' or to watch out for diabetes, or to lose weight to prevent diabetes, and patients will misunderstand and think they are already diabetic."

Ernsberger sees much of this as good news, "because far fewer people are going undiagnosed. Treatments for Type 2 diabetes have improved tremendously, and most cases can be controlled through a combination of pills, healthier diet and regular exercise. So far, there is no evidence that fasting blood sugar levels have increased in the population."

As for claims that we are for the first time seeing Type 2 diabetes among children, and especially inner-city minority children, Ernsberger points out that childhood Type 2 diabetes "has been known for decades, but no one ever determined its prevalence until recently. Until recently, epidemiological studies focused on white suburban middle-aged men and women, while children, minorities and inner-city residents were ignored." Indeed, even as organizations such as the Centers for Disease Control have issued warnings about a supposed epidemic of Type 2 diabetes, their own statistics indicate that rates of the disease hardly altered over the last decade, despite the obesity "epidemic." (According to the CDC, over the course of the 1990s the incidence of Type 2 diabetes increased from 8.2 to 8.6 percent, while the obesity rate rose by 61%.)

Furthermore . . . several recent studies indicate that the key to avoiding Type 2 diabetes is not to try to lose weight (indeed there is much evidence that dieters are far more prone to the disease than average), but rather to make lifestyle changes in regard to activity levels and dietary content that greatly reduce the risk of contracting the disease, whether or not such changes lead to any weight loss. . . .

[Recent weight loss] often correlates with increased mortality risk, even when one controls for smoking and preexisting disease. The reasons why are not well understood. Nevertheless certain aspects of the medical literature are suggestive, in particular studies that indicate weight cycling (a.k.a. yo-yo dieting) is a major factor in the development of clogged arteries, congestive heart failure, hypertension, and other serious health problems. Indeed, dieters as a group run up to double the risk of developing cardiovascular disease and Type 2 diabetes when compared to "overweight" people who do not diet. This may be a result of the fact that dieting often leads to bingeing, which is extremely unhealthy, since it is driven by cravings for high-fat, high-sugar foods (indeed, the more often a person diets, the stronger these cravings become). These foods, when consumed by people who have been depriving themselves of adequate calorie intake, are quickly metabolized into visceral body fat, which is far more dangerous to health than subcutaneous fat. (Large people who do not diet tend to have high percentages of subcutaneous fat, but low percentages of visceral fat. Also, physical activity burns visceral fat very quickly, which helps explain why, as we shall see, activity levels are far more important to health than weight.)

What about claims that even small amounts of weight loss have beneficial health effects for people suffering from hypertension and Type 2 diabetes? On closer inspection, these claims are based on studies in which sedentary people with poor dietary habits became physically active and began eating a more nutritious diet. Such studies indicate that the health benefits of these sorts of lifestyle changes are almost wholly independent of whether these changes led to any significant weight loss. As Ernsberger notes, statements to the effect that even a 10% weight reduction can be highly beneficial actually "prove that body weight is nearly irrelevant to health. People who weigh 300 pounds and then lose 10% of their body weight on a balanced low-fat diet rich in fruits and vegetables are still 'morbidly obese,' but their blood sugar, blood pressure and cholesterol have all improved." He points out that "physiologically there is little difference between a 270-pound person maintaining a healthy

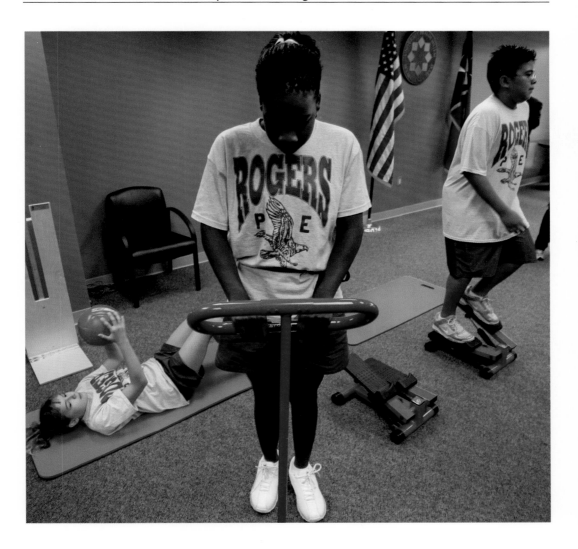

Students at Rogers Middle School in San Antonio, Texas, exercise as part of a program aimed at reducing childhood obesity. (**AP Images.**)

lifestyle and a 110-pound person. How then can we say that body fat is so deadly? Doesn't this prove that it is lifestyle, not body fat, that is crucial?"

The prevalence of—and the devastating health effects that sometimes follow from—yo-yo dieting, along with the high mortality rates found among people who are just a few pounds under what the government and the health establishment have mischaracterized as an "ideal weight," both provide powerful evidence for the proposition that attempting to lose weight causes far more damage to our health than maintaining even very high weight levels. And even if it were true that heavier people would be healthier if they lost weight, this would still be irrelevant for the purposes of public health policy if most people who intentionally lose weight then regain it, as in fact they do.

Chromium Supplements Treat Diabetes

Densie Webb

In this article Densie Webb, a writer with *Environmental Nutrition*, reports on a panel of experts at a summit, "Chromium in Health and Disease." At the summit the experts shared the results of their research on the medical effects of chromium. The article notes that people with both type 1 and type 2 diabetes experience an abnormally large loss of chromium through their urine. Chromium supplements provide a measurable reduction in insulin resistance. Other research suggests that chromium lowers blood sugar among those with type 1 diabetes.

Leading experts on the mineral chromium came together in early April [2003] in Boston for a summit titled, "Chromium in Health and Disease." *EN* [*Environmental Nutrition*] was there to report on the latest research.

SOURCE: Densie Webb, "Chromium Connections: Promising Health Roles Surface at Expert Summit," *Environmental Nutrition*, vol. 26, June 2003, p. 1. Copyright © 2003 Environmental Nutrition, Inc. Reproduced by permission.

Experts Share the Benefits of Chromium

At the conference, researchers revealed some exciting new health roles for chromium and reinforced some old ones. Among the most important: chromium's role in preventing and controlling diabetes and heart disease

Nutritional supplements that include heavy metals such as chromium may help in the battle against diabetes. (**AP Images.**)

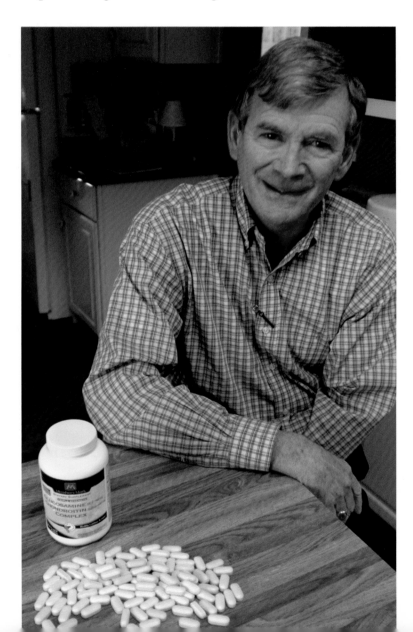

and, more surprisingly, as a possible treatment for depression.

New Data for Diabetes

Researchers discovered some time ago that chromium boosts the activity of insulin, which in turn aids the body's ability to metabolize glucose. It is only natural, then, to project that chromium might benefit people with diabetes. Now, researchers have also linked chromium to a reduction in insulin resistance, often the forerunner to type 2 diabetes.

The link is clear. Conference speakers pointed out that people with type 2 diabetes lose almost twice as much chromium in their urine and have lower levels of the mineral in their blood than people without diabetes.

William Cefalu, M.D., of the University of Vermont College of Medicine, presented findings from a well-controlled trial of people at risk for type 2 diabetes. Those given 1,000 micrograms a day of chromium picolinate experienced significant improvement in insulin sensitivity compared to those getting a placebo. Cefalu is currently involved in a new six-month study of people already diagnosed with type 2 diabetes.

"So far," he said, "I'm seeing 100% response in those who are obese, in terms of a positive effect on blood glucose." Richard Anderson, Ph.D., a longtime chromium researcher with the U.S. Department of Agriculture (USDA), said research clearly shows that chromium supplements can improve blood sugar control even beyond the benefits of glucose-lowering medications. He insists, "Even people with type 1 diabetes show improvement with chromium supplements."

Key to Heart Disease in Toenails?

Researchers from Johns Hopkins University and Harvard's School of Public Health reported on similar research from the U.S., Europe and Israel. Their findings

FAST FACT

A number of clinical studies have shown that daily chromium picolinate supplements can enhance insulin function and improve blood sugar metabolism.

strongly suggest a role for chromium in heart health. In two separate studies, chromium levels in toenails (believed to be a good indicator of chromium status in the body) were measured in men and compared to the number of heart attacks they had experienced. In both studies, the less chromium present in their toenails, the greater their risk of heart attack.

"The connection was strongest among men who were overweight," said Harvard's Eric Rimm, Sc.D. The findings reinforce the idea that there may be connections among chromium status, insulin resistance, diabetes and heart disease.

New Role in Depression?

The newest and perhaps the most exciting finding of the conference was the revelation that chromium may play a role in treating "atypical" depression, which constitutes 22% of all depression. It includes any depression that does not meet criteria for other specific depressive disorders. It often manifests itself during the teen years as a social phobia or sensitivity to rejection.

Jonathan Davidson, M.D., of Duke University Medical Center in Durham, North Carolina, presented the findings of a well-controlled study in which he gave 15 patients suffering from depression either a placebo or 400 micrograms of chromium picolinate a day. During the eight-week study, those getting chromium were increased to 600 micrograms.

The dramatic results? Of those getting chromium, 60% experienced relief from symptoms—in some cases rapidly. "This compares to antidepressant medications, which have a 40% to 50% rate of success and typically come with side effects that many patients find intolerable," said Davidson. A larger trial to further test chromium's effectiveness in treating depression is planned.

What About Safety?

Earlier laboratory studies have suggested the possibility of genetic damage with large doses of chromium picolinate. However, chromium has generally been considered one of the safest minerals. Scientific panels in both the U.S. and Britain have found no evidence of harmful effects, even at extremely high doses of up to 10,000 micrograms a day of the picolinate form.

The USDA's Anderson and John Hathcock, Ph.D., an expert on vitamin and mineral safety at the Council for Responsible Nutrition, a supplement industry trade group, reviewed the safety studies done to date. Their conclusion, they told conference attendees, is that chromium has a low toxicity. They found no studies that documented any consistent negative effects of chromium in people or animals. That includes the results of a clinical study that specifically tested for DNA damage in people taking 1,000 micrograms of chromium picolinate a day.

Where to Find the Most Chromium

This odd collection of foods and drinks represents the best information available about the richest sources of chromium:

American cheese	Brewer's Yeast	Orange juice
Apples	Broccoli	Red wine
Beef	Coffee	Tea
Banana	Green beans	Whole-wheat bread

Source: Denise Webb, "Chromium Connections: Promising Health Roles Surface at Expert Summit." *Environmental Nutrition* 26.6, June 2003.

Time to Take a Supplement?

The question then, is whether you should increase your chromium intake in hopes of fending off diabetes, heart disease and possibly depression. The experts at the summit weren't making any promises, of course, but they were optimistic that good chromium nutrition might help defend against these diseases. It may not be coincidence that chromium levels in the body decrease with age, dropping by about 25% to 40% as the risk for metabolic syndrome, diabetes and heart disease increases. This increased need, at a time of decreased availability, makes seniors more vulnerable to chromium depletion.

Flying in the face of these facts, the Institute of Medicine, which only recently made specific recommendations for chromium, put the recommended intake for people over 50 at 20 micrograms a day for women and 30 for men, inexplicably lower than its recommendations of 25 (women) and 35 (men) for younger people.

Chromium is present in a lot of foods, but most provide only one to two micrograms per serving, and dietary chromium is poorly absorbed. Virtually all of the chromium studies that have triggered a positive response used supplements, not foods. . . .

Not everyone should run out and buy chromium supplements; the potential for benefit seems to be greatest for overweight people at risk for diabetes and heart disease. If you're at risk for either condition, discuss taking chromium supplements with your doctor. Most of the evidence suggests it won't hurt and it could possibly help.

Look for supplements of chromium picolinate, the most stable and best absorbed form, at a dose of 200 to 1,000 micrograms a day, the amounts used in research. A ConsumerLab.com review of chromium picolinate supplements found most brands tested to be reliable.

Chromium Supplements Do Not Treat Diabetes

Paula R. Trumbo and Kathleen C. Ellwood

The U. S. Food and Drug Administration (FDA) must approve health-related claims made for food or food supplements. This article is written by Paula R. Trumbo and Kathleen C. Ellwood, both researchers with the FDA. In it they discuss whether chromium food supplements can reduce the risk of acquiring type 2 diabetes. Trumbo and Ellwood reject a number of studies testing the relationship between chromium and diabetes. These studies have inconclusive results or improper testing methods, they argue. They conclude that the relationship between chromium and type 2 diabetes remains uncertain.

The relationship between chromium intake and glucose metabolism was first reported in the 1950s, when chromium-containing brewer's yeast was reported to prevent diabetes in laboratory animals. Patients

SOURCE: Paula R. Trumbo and Kathleen C. Ellwood, "Chromium Picolinate Intake and Risk of Type 2 Diabetes," *Nutrition Reviews*, vol. 64, August 2006, pp. 357–63. Copyright © 2006 International Life Sciences Institute. Reproduced by permission.

who were deficient in chromium were reported to exhibit symptoms or complications of type 2 diabetes (e.g., peripheral neuropathy, impaired glucose removal, and elevated plasma free fatty acids). The provision of chromium to these patients eliminated the symptoms and complications. While chromium's metabolic role in glucose metabolism is not fully understood, it has been hypothesized that it serves as a cofactor for insulin action.

Health Claims Must Be Substantiated

The Nutrition Labeling and Education Act (NLEA) of 1990 authorized the US Food and Drug Administration (FDA) to allow statements on conventional foods and dietary supplements that describe the relationship between a substance (food or food component) and a disease (e.g., coronary heart disease, cancer, or type 2 diabetes) or health-related condition. This relationship is called a health claim.

A health-related condition (e.g., hypertension) is a condition that is essentially indistinguishable from a disease (e.g., coronary heart disease) and/or is a surrogate marker for risk of a specific disease (e.g., serum cholesterol levels for coronary heart disease). Health claims were first authorized under the significant scientific agreement (SSA) standard, a rigorous standard that requires a high level of confidence in the validity of a substance-disease relationship. Due to court decisions dealing with health claims for dietary supplements that raised First Amendment issues, and a major initiative introduced by FDA in 2003, qualified health claims were established for the labeling of conventional foods and dietary supplements. When credible evidence falls short of the SSA standard, then health claims with qualifying language about the level of scientific evidence (qualified health claims) are issued through letters of enforcement discretion. SSA and qualified health claims pertain to disease risk reduction in the US population or a target subgroup (e.g., women or the elderly) who do not have the disease that is the subject of the claim. . . .

Chromium Picolinate and Blood Sugar Concentration

FDA identified 13 studies evaluating the effect of chromium picolinate supplementation on blood glucose concentrations. Eight of these studies were not further reviewed because scientific conclusions could not be drawn from them for the following reasons. Walker et al. did not provide the data within the report; therefore, the agency was not able to evaluate the reliability or the statistical interpretation of the data. In three of the studies, the subjects were already diagnosed with diabetes.

A diabetic man receives counseling from a dietitian. (**AP Images.**)

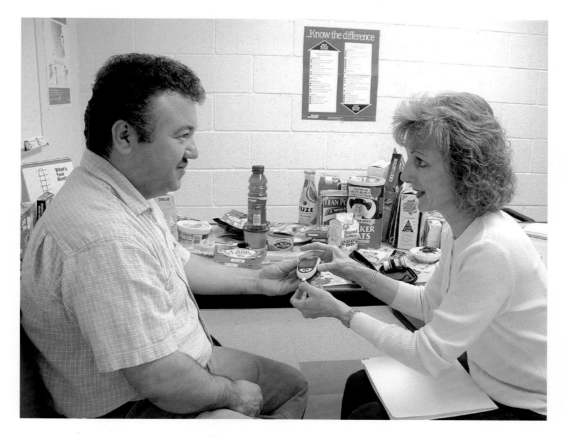

Two studies did not include a control group. Statistical analyses were not conducted between the chromium picolinate and control group in two studies. Volpe et al. conducted a 12-week, randomized study that provided obese US women . . . 400 mg/d of chromium as chromium picolinate. This study was found to be of moderate methodological quality.

There was no statistically significant difference in fasting blood sugar (FBS) or oral glucose tolerance test (OGTT) between the chromium picolinate and the placebo group. Boyd et al. was a 13-week, non-randomized study in which healthy US men and women . . . were given either a placebo or 1 g/d chromium picolinate.

This study was found to be of moderate methodological quality. There was no statistically significant beneficial effect of chromium picolinate on FBS or OGTT compared with the placebo control group.

A 12-week, randomized study by Joseph et al. was conducted on US men and women who were healthy or had glucose intolerance. This study was found to be of moderate methodological quality. Subjects . . . received either a placebo or 924 mg/d of chromium as chromium picolinate and underwent resistance training twice weekly. There was no statistically significant beneficial effect of chromium picolinate on FBS compared with the control group.

Frauchiger et al. was a single-dose, crossover design study in which young Swiss men . . . were provided a placebo or 400 or 800 mg of chromium as chromium picolinate 30 minutes prior to the consumption of a test meal. This study was found to be of moderate methodological quality. There was no statistically significant beneficial effect . . . OGTT when either 400 or 800 mg of chromium picolinate was consumed.

FAST FACT

According to the American Diabetes Association (ADA), only patients with very low chromium levels experience problems; for most people, chromium supplements offer no known benefits.

Cefalu et al. was a double-blind, randomized study in which subjects at high risk for diabetes . . . were provided a placebo or 1000 mg/d of chromium picolinate for 8 months. There was no statistically beneficial effect of chromium picolinate on OGTT compared with the control group.

Other Forms of Chromium

FDA identified 29 studies evaluating the effect of other forms of chromium on blood sugar levels. Four of these studies did not include a control group for comparing the relative effect of chromium. Nine studies did not conduct statistical analyses between the control and chromium group. One study was conducted on hypoglycemic patients to determine if chromium chloride had an effect on blood glucose levels. The purpose of that study, however, was to determine if chromium chloride would increase low blood glucose to normal levels, and therefore it did not address the proposed claim for a reduction in risk of elevated blood glucose levels. Three studies were conducted in malnourished children in Jordan, Turkey, and Egypt. Nutrient status and metabolism can be severely altered when an individual is malnourished. For example, malnutrition can result in lower blood glucose and insulin levels, and therefore the effect of a nutrient, such as chromium, on blood sugar levels can be very different than the effect of the same nutrient on healthy, well-nourished individuals.

Thus, scientific conclusions about the effect of other forms of chromium on blood sugar levels in the general US population could not be drawn from these 17 studies. There have been 11 studies on healthy subjects, one study on individuals with glucose intolerance, and one study on both healthy subjects and those with hyperglycemia that evaluated the effect of other forms of chromium (chromium chloride and chromium nicotinate) on blood glucose levels. These studies were found to be of moderate to high methodological quality. None of the 12 studies in healthy subjects showed a significant beneficial effect of chromium supplementation on FBS and/or OGTT. The two studies in individuals with glucose intolerance showed no significant beneficial effect of chromium supplementation on FBS. One of the two studies showed a statistically significant benefit for OGTT over a 4-hour period in hyperglycemic individuals.

Chromium Picolinate and Type 2 Diabetes

No studies were identified by FDA that evaluated the effect of chromium picolinate supplementation on the incidence of type 2 diabetes. Thus, the only evidence to support a relationship between chromium picolinate intake and risk of type 2 diabetes are the studies discussed above that measured the effect of chromium picolinate intake on two surrogate endpoints: insulin resistance and blood sugar levels. . . .

Little Evidence of Blood Sugar Reduction

In summary, there was one intervention study that showed a beneficial effect of chromium picolinate intake on risk of insulin resistance. One other intervention study that provided chromium chloride showed no beneficial effect on insulin resistance. None of the five intervention studies showed a statistically significant beneficial effect of chromium picolinate on FBS and/or OGTT. Furthermore, none of the 10 intervention studies using other forms of chromium showed a beneficial effect on FBS or OGTT in individuals with normal glucose tolerance.

Based on FDA's evidence-based review, the agency concluded that there is very limited credible evidence for a qualified health claim for chromium picolinate and reduced risk of insulin resistance, and therefore reduced risk of type 2 diabetes. The findings of Cefalu et al. have

Symptoms of Chromium Deficiency

✓ Fasting hyperglycemia (too much blood sugar)
✓ Hypoglycemia (too little blood sugar)
✓ Decreased insulin receptors
✓ Decreased insulin binding
✓ Decreased lean body mass
✓ Elevated percentage of body fat
✓ Peripheral neuropathy
✓ Fatigue and/or anxiety

Source: The Nutrition Solution.

not been replicated, and replication of scientific findings is important to substantiate results. For these reasons, FDA concluded that the existence of a relationship between chromium picolinate intake and reduced risk of either insulin resistance or type 2 diabetes is highly uncertain.

On August 25, 2005, FDA issued a letter of enforcement discretion for the labeling of dietary supplements with the following qualified health claim: "One small study suggests that chromium picolinate may reduce the risk of insulin resistance, and therefore possibly may reduce the risk of type 2 diabetes. FDA concludes, however, that the existence of such a relationship between chromium picolinate and either insulin resistance or type 2 diabetes is highly uncertain." The agency concluded that there was no credible evidence to suggest that chromium picolinate intake may reduce the risk of elevated blood glucose levels.

Herbal Remedies Can Help Control Blood Sugar

Dave Tuttle

Dave Tuttle writes for *Life Extension*, a publication of the Life Extension Foundation. The Life Extension Foundation is a nonprofit organization that researches ways to extend the human life span. In this article he discusses the ways that cinnamon and coffee berries help the body improve its ability to produce insulin. He cites research by the U.S. Department of Agriculture and Iowa State University that demonstrates the benefits of cinnamon. He describes other research showing that cinnamon could lower cholesterol. Tuttle says that coffee berries and to a lesser extent coffee beans contain nutrients that help lower the risk of acquiring type 2 diabetes.

Cinnamon has been used for several thousand years in traditional Ayurvedic and Greco-European medical systems. Native to tropical southern India and Sri Lanka, the bark of this evergreen tree is used to

SOURCE: Dave Tuttle, "Controlling Blood Sugar with Cinnamon and Coffee Berry," *Life Extension, Collector's Edition*, 2006, p. 20–2. Reproduced by permission.

PERSPECTIVES ON DISEASES AND DISORDERS

manage conditions such as nausea, bloating, flatulence, and anorexia. It is also one of the world's most common spices, used to flavor everything from oatmeal and apple cider to cappuccino.

Recent research has revealed, however, that regular use of cinnamon can promote healthy glucose metabolism. A study performed at the US Department of Agriculture's Beltsville Human Nutrition Research Center isolated insulin-enhancing complexes in cinnamon that are involved in preventing or alleviating glucose intolerance and diabetes. Three water-soluble polyphenol polymers were found to have beneficial biological activity, increasing insulin-dependent glucose metabolism by roughly 20-fold in vitro. The nutrients displayed significant antioxidant activity as well, as did other phytochemicals found in cinnamon, such as epicatechin, phenol, and tannin. Moreover, scientists at Iowa State University determined that these polyphenol polymers are able to up-regulate the expression of genes involved in activating the cell membrane's insulin receptors, thus increasing glucose uptake and lowering blood glucose levels.

Animal Experiments

These benefits of cinnamon have been confirmed in animal experiments. For example, when rats were given two different doses of an oral cinnamon supplement for three weeks, glucose infusion into their cells more than doubled, even with the lower dose studied. The extract improved insulin action by enhancing the insulin-signaling pathway in skeletal muscle, resulting in increased glucose uptake.

Cinnamon can even help control the negative effects of a diet high in fructose, a simple sugar. When rats were fed large amounts of fructose for three weeks with or without the addition of cinnamon extract to their drinking water, the cinnamon extract improved the glucose infusion rate in the fructose-fed animals so much that it equaled that of control rats eating a standard chow diet. According to the study authors, this suggests that the early use of cinnamon could prevent the development of insulin resistance in those who consume abundant fructose sugar.

Cinnamon and Heart Disease

Because the incidence of cardiovascular disease is increased up to fourfold in type II diabetics, researchers have sought out nutrients that can simultaneously im-

A worker picks coffee beans near Palmares, Costa Rica. Natural products such as coffee berries and cinnamon have been shown to lower the risk of developing type 2 diabetes. (AP Images.)

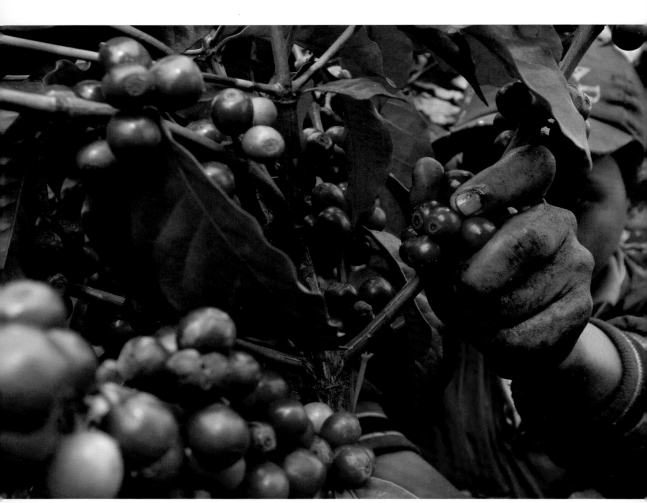

prove glucose metabolism and lipid levels. In a recent study published in *Diabetes Care*, cinnamon proved to be such a dual-action agent. Sixty adults (30 men, 30 women) with type II diabetes were divided into six groups. The first three groups consumed one, three, or six grams of cinnamon daily, while the other three groups consumed equivalent numbers of placebo capsules.

The spice or placebo was consumed for 40 days, followed by a 20-day washout period. After the initial 40-day period, all three levels of cinnamon reduced mean fasting serum glucose levels by 18-29%. The one-gram dose also reduced triglyceride levels by 18%, low-density lipoprotein (LDL) by 7%, and total cholesterol by 12%. Higher doses of cinnamon produced even greater reductions in triglycerides, LDL, and total cholesterol.

Even better, these decreases persisted throughout the 20-day washout period. While glucose and triglyceride levels increased modestly during the washout period compared to day-40 levels, they remained below the levels recorded before cinnamon supplementation began. Meanwhile, LDL and total cholesterol levels continued to decline throughout the 20 days after cinnamon use stopped. This study suggests that cinnamon has sustained effects, so the benefits should continue even if a dose is occasionally missed. The results also suggest doses of one gram or more are likely to be beneficial in controlling blood glucose and lipid levels.

Cinnamon May Stimulate Insulin

Cinnamon thus appears to be one of the most powerful nutrients available for improving glucose metabolism. USDA researchers at the Beltsville center studied the effects of 49 herbs, spices, and medicinal plant extracts on glucose utilization in the fat cells of rats.

They found that cinnamon was the most bioactive product, followed by witch hazel, green and black teas, and allspice. The active phytochemicals in cinnamon were determined to be the polyphenols. Another Beltsville study found that cinnamon potentiated insulin activity more than threefold.

Coffee Berries Cut Diabetes Risks

Coffee is one of the world's most popular beverages, yet most people know very little about the fruit that produces coffee beans. Grown in mountainous tropical climates, the brightly colored fruit ripens into a glowing red berry that is usually harvested by hand. The berry's exterior is discarded and the bean is dried and processed. Roasting normally occurs in the country where the beverage will be consumed.

However, as with many fruits, most of the powerful nutritional benefits of coffee are found in the whole fruit itself, not just in the seed (or bean). Nature evolved the cherry of the coffee shrub to withstand intense ultraviolet radiation found at mountainous elevations. As a result, whole coffee fruit is loaded with beneficial antioxidants and other powerful plant nutrients that are partially destroyed during the separation and roasting processes of conventional coffee production.

This nutrient-rich coffee fruit has been relegated to virtual obscurity because it quickly deteriorates during normal coffee harvesting. Now, however, a patent-pending technology has been developed that preserves the whole coffee fruit, eliminating the potential for toxicity and making it possible to develop supplements that contain all of the nutrients naturally found in the fruit.

The coffee berry contains some well-studied phytochemicals such as chlorogenic acid, caffeic acid, ferulic acid, and quinic acid. These nutrients have recently been shown to help quench free radicals, provide cardiovascular benefits, and reduce cholesterol oxidation. How-

> **FAST FACT**
>
> Herbs used to treat diabetes have been known to help lower blood sugar levels, improve the body's ability to metabolize and respond to insulin, and support pancreas function.

ever, some of the coffee berry's most impressive effects can be seen in blood glucose management.

Studies Confirm the Benefits of Coffee

Three studies have shown that coffee consumption helps reduce the risk of type II diabetes. In an analysis of more than 17,000 Dutch men and women, the more coffee a person drank, the lower the incidence of diabetes. Consuming three to four cups a day decreased the risk by 23%, while persons drinking more than seven cups daily cut their risk in half.

A study among middle-aged Finnish men and women confirmed these results. The Finns drink more coffee per capita than any nation in the world, so its impact on their public health could be dramatic. After controlling for numerous variables, this study found that consuming three to four cups a day reduced diabetes risk by 24%.

Those consuming 10 or more cups lowered their risk by 61%. The scientists suggested that this protective effect is partially due to the inhibition of glucose-6-phosphatase activity by chlorogenic acid, since glucose-6-phosphatase is widely considered a significant factor in the abnormally high rates of hepatic glucose production observed in the

Sales of Cinnamon to Treat Diabetes

Cinnamon	Current Dollars	Year Ago Dollars	$%Change
Conventional Food/Drug/ Mass Marketers	$1,036,179	$67,532	1434.4%
Natural Supermarkets	$1,334,567	$277,534	380.9%
Total	$3,906,019	$345,066	1032.0%

Source: SPINscan Natural and Conventional Channels.

diabetic state. Consequently, they believe that reduced glucose-6-phosphatase hydrolysis can lower glucose output, leading to decreased plasma glucose concentrations.

Chlorogenic acid also has an antagonistic effect on glucose transporters at the intestinal stage, and has been shown to influence the secretion of two gastrointestinal peptides known for their glucose-lowering effects. These various mechanisms may explain why coffee can produce such a dramatic decrease in the incidence of diabetes.

Another study of coffee consumption explored the relative benefits of caffeinated versus decaffeinated coffee. This analysis examined the intake patterns of more than 41,000 men and nearly 85,000 women participating in the Health Professionals Follow-up Study and the Nurses' Health Study. Due to the different start dates for these investigations, the men were followed for 13 years and the women for 18 years. While the researchers found correlations between regular caffeinated coffee and diabetes that were similar to those of previous studies, they also discovered a lesser, but still significant, relationship between decaffeinated coffee and disease incidence. After controlling for several variables, men who drank one to three cups of decaffeinated coffee daily reduced their risk by 9%, while those drinking four or more cups a day lowered it by 26%.

Women experienced a slightly smaller reduction in risk than men. Tea drinkers saw no decrease in their risk for diabetes. While caffeine intake is associated with a decreased risk of type II diabetes, intake of decaffeinated coffee can still cut your chances of developing diabetes. For those who wish to avoid stimulants like caffeine, this is good news indeed.

Herbal Remedies Are Not Necessarily Safe

C. Day

Author C. Day works for the Diabetes Research Group of Aston University in Great Britain. In the following article Day explores the use of a variety of herbal supplements to treat diabetes. Noting that many Americans and Britons use nonconventional medicines, the author says that over one thousand herbal treatments have been claimed to help in the treatment of diabetes. Some traditional remedies have been used for centuries, according to Day. The author states that using herbal medicine can be dangerous. Some, including cinnamon, may have toxic properties. The side effects of long-term use of large doses are unknown.

A ccording to the USA National Center for Complementary and Alternative Medicine (NCCAM), more than 75% of American adults have used some kind of complementary or alternative medicine, whilst a prevalence figure of 20% has been suggested for use of non-conventional medicine in the UK. Our own occasional surveys in the past 20 years in diabetes outpatient clinics and primary care centres in Birmingham [UK] found that the number of patients who admit to ever using non-conventional therapies has remained at about 3%. These patients generally used herbal medicines: mostly those that were currently receiving acclaim in the popular press, but in general the remedies were not for the treatment of diabetes or its complications. Patients of Afro-Caribbean and Indo-Asian origin were more likely to use herbal remedies, with cerasee and karela (wild and cultivated varieties of *Momordica charantia*, respectively) being considered of benefit in the treatment of diabetes. However, these remedies were generally only used intermittently (e.g. to improve glycaemia prior to clinic visits) and were not employed as regular treatments for diabetes.

Media attempts to undermine conventional medical practice have fuelled a market for alternative (non-conventional) remedies based on anecdotal accounts of benefits, without any recognized validation that the feted remedy is either safe or efficacious.

Several non-conventional practices have been cited for the treatment of diabetes. Common explanations to account for their reputations include pancreatic stimulation (to secrete insulin), stimulation of 'healing energy channels' (whatever they are?), promote relaxation (reduce stress hormone release) and biochemical 'balancing' (again inadvertently elaborate). The more sceptical explanations are that the therapies have a placebo effect, with any improvements due to attention received from the therapist resulting in adherence to sensible dietary and lifestyle advice.

With acupuncture, electrostimulation of the Zhongwan acupoint increased plasma insulin and plasma ß-endorphin in normal and non-insulin-dependent diabetic rats. Administration of naloxone blocked this

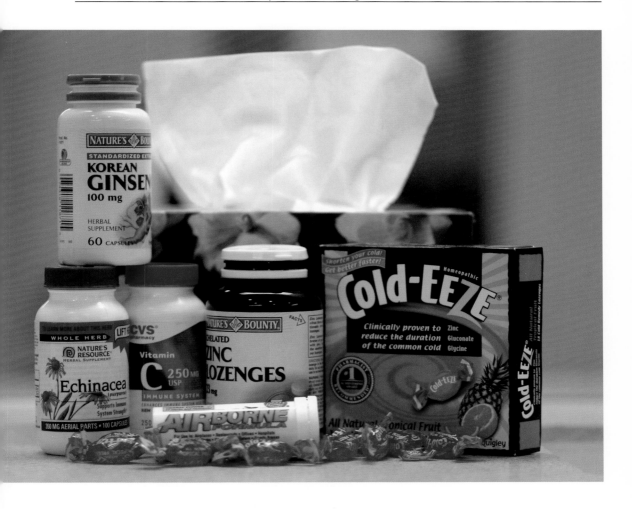

antidiabetic effect, suggesting that the effect may be mediated via endogenous opiate release, adding a further twist to debate over the role of opiates in glucose homeostasis. Interestingly, electrostimulation at non-specific sites did not improve glycaemic control, emphasizing the importance of performing acupuncture according to traditional instruction.

Most Herbal Remedies Untested

More than 1000 plants have been claimed to benefit the treatment of diabetes—there is no botanical substitute

While some have asserted the benefits of herbal medicines in treating diabetes and other ailments, many scientists have questioned their effectiveness and their long-term safety. (AP Images.)

for insulin—but few have received adequate scientific and clinical scrutiny. Whilst it is fashionable to undertake systematic database searches, this approach offers no substitute for critically reviewing the original publications. Databases should be viewed as listings of publications: they do not provide validation of either the journals or quality of material published. Abstracts often contain very positive statements, which are not justified by the methodology and/or results of the study described. This area is also complicated by a need for overlapping expertise. For example, an acceptable clinical study in a medical journal may suffer from flawed botanical taxonomy or pharmacognosy, while a study with sound 'plant medicine' may not conform to adequate criteria for a 'diabetes trial'. Nevertheless, the studies may still be accepted for publication—often in specialist journals—and archived on databases.

To validate traditional usage, it is important that plants are accurately botanically identified, collected, prepared and administered in accordance with traditional practice. Conformity of plant material allows further studies to gain more information on a potential treatment. . . .

Many different moieties and chemical groups with antidiabetic activity have been isolated from plants traditionally used to treat diabetes, but a range of factors has precluded further development into pharmaceutical products. Nevertheless it is encouraging to recall that metformin, the single most prescribed agent for the treatment of diabetes, has its origin in herbal medicine.

Herbal Remedies Used for Centuries

Diet has long been the cornerstone of diabetes treatments. The Ebers Papyrus (1550 B.C.) prescribed a diet rich in wheatgerm and ochra, both of which have subsequently been shown to exert gluco-lowering efficacy. Karela, the cultivated variety of *Momodica charantia*

Linn, a standard ingredient of the Indo-Asian diet, is often used as a treatment for diabetes. Reliable studies have shown that karela reduces hyperglycaemia in Type 2 diabetes without stimulation of insulin. This is achieved via mechanisms that inhibit hepatic glucose output and possibly to a lesser extent by altering intestinal glucose handling. Karela yielded several weakly active alkaloidal compounds, but they were deemed too toxic for pharmaceutical development. However, as a dietary adjunct, rather than a chronic medicinal treatment, karela consumption can help to control hyperglycaemia. Karela tablets are available via the internet and some Indo-Asian magazines in the UK.

> ## FAST FACT
>
> An overdose of herbs is as real and deadly as an overdose of prescription drugs.

These preparations have not been subjected to conventional pharmaceutical testing, yet some imply product endorsement based on literature references only. . . . Recently, media attention has focused on the antidiabetic properties of cinnamon, traditionally used on the Indian subcontinent. In 1981 a conference report noted that consumption of powdered cinnamon (*Cinnamomum tamala*) for a month decreased fasting plasma glucose and improved glucose tolerance in diabetic patients. Increased insulin secretion was observed 30 min after consumption of 20 g of powdered cinnamon. An insulin secretory action of cinnamon was confirmed in isolated islets and bioactive cinnamon compounds have been shown to improve insulin action in rat epididymal adipocytes upstream of phosphatidylinositol 3-kinase, suggesting benefits in treating insulin resistance.

Water-soluble polyphenol polymers isolated from cinnamon increased insulin-dependent glucose metabolism in vitro and displayed antioxidant activity. In a randomized, placebo-controlled trial in diabetic patients in Pakistan, daily consumption of 1 g, 3 g or 6 g of *Cinnamomum cassia* powder, as capsules, for 40 days followed by a 20 day washout period reduced fasting serum glucose throughout the treatment period and this benefit was still evident at the end of the washout period. Lipid parameters were also improved.

Current data suggest that cinnamon is worthy of further investigation. However, it is not advisable to recommend clinical usage of cinnamon until information is available on the effects of chronic consumption of relatively large volumes of this plant. Cinnamon, like karela, may be found to contain antidiabetic moieties with toxic properties, which preclude usage beyond standard dietary inclusion. Nevertheless, this clinical study is cited by a Louisiana-based company to support web-marketing of a 'diabetes' product containing cinnamon.

Herbal Remedies Can Be Dangerous

The dangers of herbal medicines cannot be overstated. In January 2004 the American Diabetes Association issued a position statement regarding the use of 'unproven therapies' and highlighted the need for therapeutic

Non-conventional Diabetes Therapies

Acupuncture	Aromatherapy	Biofeedback
Energy healing	Herbalism	Homeopathy
Hypnotherapy	Lifestyle diets	Massage
Osteopathy	Reflexology	Yoga

Source: C. Day, "Are Herbal Remedies of Use in Diabetes?" *Diabetic Medicine*, vol. 22, January 2005.

modalities to have established safety and efficacy. The statement also recommended that patients be asked specifically about their use of non-conventional therapies. In June 2004 the World Health Organization sounded an alarm about the unregulated and often unsafe use of non-conventional therapies and noted that in China the reporting of adverse reactions in 2002 was double the number registered for the 1990s. Herbal remedies alone may have deleterious effects or may interact with conventional medication. For example, ginseng, a traditional antidiabetic remedy with conflicting reports regarding efficacy, has been reported to decrease the anticoagulant effects of warfarin significantly. In diabetes effective remedies may increase the risk of hypoglycaemia with concurrent conventional medicines.

Death cap mushroom (*Amanita phalloides*) gained its name by causing irreversible hypoglycaemia, unripe ackee fruit (*Blighia sapida*) decreases glycaemia via potentially fatal hepatic glycogen depletion, and periwinkle (*Vinca rosa*), which is widely recommended in the treatment of diabetes, is better known for its toxic components, e.g. the anticancer alkaloids vinblastine and vincristine.

Plant remedies may be appealing as alternative or adjunctive treatments for diabetes, but natural is not necessarily safe.

Embryonic Stem Cells Are Needed for Diabetes Research

Juvenile Diabetes Research Foundation

The Juvenile Diabetes Research Foundation (JDRF) is a nonprofit foundation dedicated to finding a cure for type 1 diabetes. The following excerpt from a JDRF position paper highlights the work that led to the isolation of human embryonic stem cells in 1998, noting that the process had been completed with mouse cells some twenty years ago. The authors describe the advances in embryonic stem cell research and the social, political, and moral concerns that have been factors in the process. They compare the uses of adult and embryonic stem cells and conclude that medical science will benefit if research with the latter is continued.

Two years ago, President George W. Bush announced that U.S. federal funds could be used to support research using selected human embryonic stem cell lines. Then, as now, human embryonic stem cells—which had only been derived in the late 1990s—

SOURCE: Juvenile Diabetes Research Foundation, "Embryonic Stem Cells," September 2003. www.jdf.org.

represented significant potential for basic research to unravel the complex pathways by which cells and tissues develop, and for the development of cellular therapies for a wide range of diseases, including juvenile (type 1) diabetes. Over the course of the last two years, the potential for embryonic stem cells to provide insights and answers into the causes, treatment, and possible cures for type 1 diabetes, Parkinson's disease, and a host of other devastating illnesses has remained strong. International investigation is proceeding, as is discovery by both private industry and researchers funded by non-governmental sources. But a series of unforeseen factors have conspired to slow the pace of embryonic stem cell research in the U.S.; as a result, progress has been disappointing, at best.

The good news is that the promise of stem cell research to cure diseases such as juvenile diabetes, Parkinson's, and heart disease has only grown since 2001. In the case of type 1 diabetes, the potential for embryonic stem cell research to benefit scientific investigation into causes, treatments and cures for the disease and its complications is significant. Possible applications range from basic research in understanding the causes and triggers of diabetes, to replacement therapies utilizing beta cells derived from embryonic stem cells as a potential solution to the severe lack of donor organs for islet cell transplantation. To that end, experiments to create insulin-producing cells from mouse embryonic stem cells have been successful at several research centers in the past year. And more broadly, the National Institutes of Health (NIH) has undertaken a number of promising initiatives to encourage scientists to seize the opportunity embryonic stem cells offer by establishing programs to train investigators and provide support in working with approved stem cell lines.

FAST FACT

A 2007 survey of patients at U.S. infertility centers indicated that 60 percent of those surveyed would donate surplus embryos for stem cell research.

In spite of all these positive factors, however, the development of a robust research community focused on embryonic stem cell investigation, especially in the US, has been slowed by political issues, ethical debate, funding considerations, and the difficulty of recruiting and motivating scientists to concentrate their activities on a path not yet traveled by other researchers. Clearly, progress is being made, but just as clearly, the issues cited above have slowed the growth of stem cell research in the U.S. . . .

Stem Cell Research Is Relatively New

Stem cell research is among the more recent areas of scientific discovery. Researchers only isolated stem cells from mouse embryos some 20 years ago; but it wasn't until 1998 that scientists successfully isolated human embryonic stem cells, when research teams at the University of Wisconsin and Johns Hopkins University independently derived human pluripotent cells.

Embryonic stem cells are cells with two capacities believed to be unique: they are capable of seemingly limitless reproduction, and they can develop into any type of cell, tissue, or organ as they mature—an ability scientists describe as "pluripotency." At the same time, embryonic stem cells cannot themselves develop into a full organism. Their ability to replicate themselves indefinitely while remaining in an "undifferentiated" state means that embryonic stem cells offer a potentially unlimited source of cells for organ transplantation, and prove a model system for drug discovery and the study of human development.

Human embryonic stem cells are derived from surplus eggs that have been fertilized in vitro—in an in vitro fertilization clinic—and have then been specifically donated for research purposes with the informed consent of the donors. (It is estimated that up to 400,000 surplus eggs are currently stored in freezers in the U.S.) These "blastocysts" are typically four or five days old, and form a hollow, microscopic ball of about 150 cells. To derive

Stem Cell Differentiation

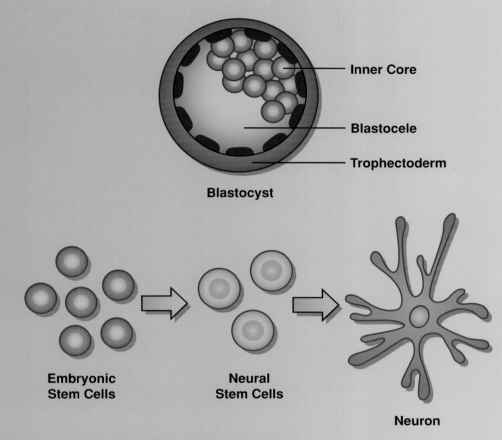

Inner Core

Blastocele

Trophectoderm

Blastocyst

Embryonic Stem Cells

Neural Stem Cells

Neuron

Source: Olympus FluoView Resource Center.

stem cells, researchers transfer the inner cell mass of a blastocyst into a laboratory culture dish that contains nutrients, or "feeder cells." Over the course of several days, the cells of the inner cell mass proliferate and begin to crowd the culture dish. The cells are removed and put into several fresh culture dishes. Stem cells that have proliferated in a cell culture for at least six months without differentiating are pluripotent, and are referred to as an embryonic stem cell line.

Embryonic Stem Cell Research Has Potential in Different Areas

There are at least three basic opportunities presented by embryonic stem cell research. First, research could lead to the development of innovative replacement or transplantation therapies for diseases such as diabetes or heart disease. In fact, embryonic stem cells are key to the increasingly promising area of regenerative medicine, which could profoundly improve our ability to prevent and cure disease. Second, the field can provide a deeper understanding of cell differentiation and development, with possible consequences for the treatment of diseases such as cancer. And third, stem cells could be used as a surrogate in the screening and testing of drugs.

Much of the research involving embryonic stem cells at this point is not specific to juvenile (type 1) diabetes, but is at a more basic-science level. Areas of intense interest include a) the study of the mechanism that maintain stem cells in an undifferentiated state; b) the development of the earliest of the three germ layers—endoderm, mesoderm, and ectoderm—from which all other tissue and organs develop; and c) the differentiation of stem cells into specific tissues and organs, such as pancreatic beta cells that produce insulin and are the key to curing type 1 diabetes.

Stem Cell Research Offers Hope for Type 1 Diabetes

The continued strong optimism for the beneficial use of stem cells is underscored by recent progress in a number of areas, including juvenile diabetes. For example, stem cells have been successfully directed towards the production of specific nervous tissue: Transplanted neural stem cells have been shown to differentiate into mature neurons to replace cells in the damaged brains of animal models of diseases such as Parkinson's. The injection of human stem cells into the fluid around the spinal cord of paralyzed rats clearly improved the animals' ability to control their hind limbs by developing into nerve cells, and by creating an environment that protected and aided existing neurons. And the transplantation of stem cells— or cardiomyocytes derived from stem cells—into damaged hearts is becoming an increasingly promising strategy for the treatment of heart disease and the restoration of heart function.

Some experiments have suggested that a small number of certain adult stem cell types may also be pluripotent—they can develop into other cell types. Adult stem cells are unspecialized cells found among differentiated cells in a tissue or organ that are capable of renewing themselves and differentiating to yield the major specialized cell types of the tissue or organ. The primary roles of adult stem cells are to maintain and repair the tissue in which they are found. Unlike embryonic stem cells, which are defined by their origin (the inner cell mass of the blastocyst), the origin of adult stem cells in mature tissues is unknown.

However, there is little evidence so far of a wide array of human adult stem cells that can differentiate into multiple tissue types. In fact, most available evidence indicates that adult stem cells do not possess the same capacity to give rise to any cell type as embryonic stem cells do. For example, even the most promising adult stem cell study did not differentiate adult stem cells into beta cells, the type relevant to treating type 1 diabetes. As a result, restricting research on embryonic stem cells and relying solely on adult stem cell studies would severely hamper medical progress, and virtually all stem cell scientists believe research should be pursued with both embryonic and adult stem cell types.

Success with Adult Stem Cells Reduces the Need for Embryonic Stem Cells Diabetes Research

William J. Cromie

William J. Cromie is a writer with the *Harvard University Gazette*. In the following article he details the breakthrough research by Denise Faustman, a professor at Harvard Medical School. Cromie describes how Faustman used adult stem cells from diabetic mice to rebuild their immune systems, which allowed them to restore normal insulin production. The long-term possibilities, Cromie reports, are not known, but the procedure offers hope for people with diabetes as well as other diseases.

The permanent reversal of Type 1 diabetes in mice may end the wrenching debate over harvesting stem cells from the unborn to treat adult diseases. Researchers at Harvard Medical School killed cells responsible for the diabetes, then the animals' adult stem

SOURCE: William J. Cromie, "Adult Stem Cells Effect a Cure," *Harvard University Gazette*, August 16, 2001. Copyright © 2002 by the President and Fellows of Harvard College. Reproduced by permission.

cells took over and regenerated missing cells needed to produce insulin and eliminate the disease.

"It should be possible to use the same method to reverse Type 1 diabetes in humans," says Denise Faustman, the associate professor of medicine who leads the research. Setting up a trial for patients has already begun [as of 2001] at Massachusetts General Hospital in Boston. Type 1 diabetes is an "autoimmune" disease in which the body's blood cells attack its own organs and tissues. Such maladies include rheumatoid arthritis, multiple sclerosis, lupus, and more than 50 other ailments. Faustman believes that many of them may be similarly cured by poisoning the offending cells and letting adult stem cells regrow replacement organs.

Adult Stem Cells Repair Damaged Organs

"Once the disease is out of the way, adult stem cells regenerate normal organs and tissues," Faustman says. "What is more, we should be able to replace damaged organs and tissues by using adult stem cells, thus eliminating, at least temporarily, the need to harvest and transplant stem cells from embryos and fetuses. Of course, it will take years before we know for sure if we can do this in humans."

Stem cells from embryos have the ability to grow into all other types of cells. They may be able to mature into brain cells to repair damage from strokes, Alzheimer's and Parkinson's diseases; into heart cells to heal the ravages of heart attacks; and into organs to replace those ruined by cancer.

But problems exist in getting such cells to mature into a specific type of cell and to home in on a specific place. There's also the problem of stopping them from growing once the repair is made. Uncontrolled growth may lead to tumors.

The existence of adult stem cells raises the question of why the body doesn't use them on a regular basis to heal

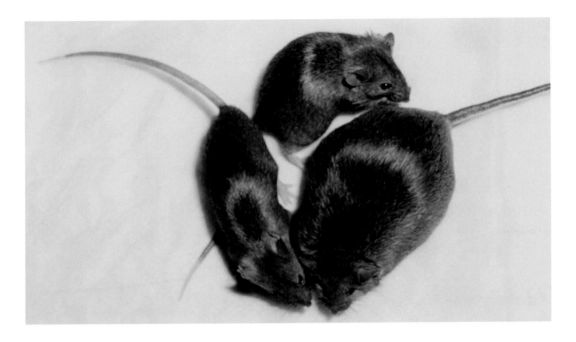

Successful trials using adult stem cells of mice to reverse their type 1 diabetes has offered the hope that embryonic stem cells may not be needed. **(AP Images.)**

itself. It may be because adult stem-cell populations are small and need some sort of outside stimulation. There's recent evidence that additional adult cells injected into mice start to repair heart attack and stroke damage.

In the diabetes experiments, cells that attack insulin-producing islet cells in the pancreas were destroyed. The researchers intended to follow up the killings with transplants of healthy islet cells but, to their surprise, this turned out to be unnecessary because adult stem cells took over the work. "It was a miracle that we didn't expect," Faustman comments.

Finding a Missing Connection

An estimated 16 million people have diabetes in the United States. About 10 percent of these patients suffer from Type 1, which used to be called juvenile diabetes because it commonly appears between ages 10 and 16. Type 1 diabetics cannot make insulin to convert blood sugars into energy, so they must inject themselves daily with the hormone to survive. New cases have tripled in the United States in the past 50 years.

Type 2, formerly called adult-onset diabetes, usually occurs gradually after age 40, and often can be managed by diet and exercise. The two types together are the leading cause of kidney failure, adult blindness, and limb amputation, as well as major risk factors for heart disease, strokes, and birth defects.

Faustman isn't sure if her technique will work with Type 2 diabetes. "We really don't know if replacing the islet cells will do the job," she says. "Some experts think that the resistance to insulin comes from outside the pancreas. There's also the possibility that Type 2 diabetics used up their stem cells at a faster rate," which decreases their repair capacity.

> **FAST FACT**
>
> A study at Canada's University of Alberta showed that insulin-producing cells derived from embryonic stem cells are not the "beta cells" required to reverse diabetes.

The Harvard—Massachusetts General Hospital team believes they can move from mice to humans because the same defective pathways exist in both species. "We always begin our projects with human cells," Faustman explains. "When we observe something important but can't experiment with patients, we go to mice."

Cancer and AIDS Research Applied to Diabetes

The defective pathway in both humans and mice has been known for years. It's been well-studied in cancer and AIDS research, but everyone missed its connection to autoimmune disease until Faustman's lab hit upon it. The defect involves a genetic mutation that causes white blood cells to attack the insulin-producing cells. It's as if the body rejects part of itself because it cannot tell the difference between normal cells and foreign invaders like viruses or bacteria. Faustman's team found they could destroy the offending cells with drugs.

When given to the mice, a compound known as CFA boosted the production of another substance known as tumor necrosis factor-alpha (TNF). Years ago, researchers tested TNF as a cancer drug, then as an AIDS treatment, but have abandoned it since. TNF wiped out cells that couldn't tell self from nonself, but this was believed to be only a temporary respite. Everyone thought it could only

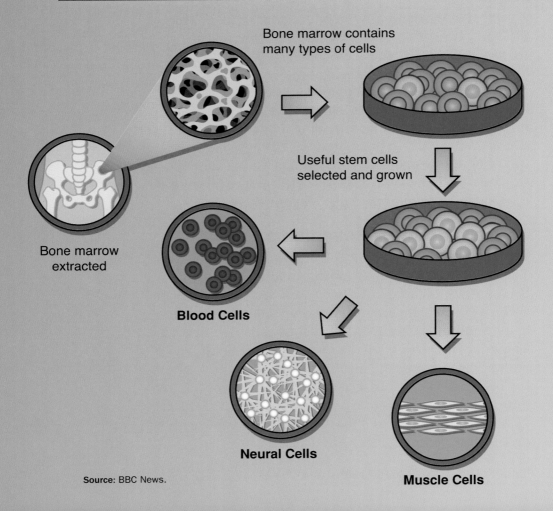

Applications of Bone Marrow Stem Cells

Bone marrow contains many types of cells

Bone marrow extracted

Useful stem cells selected and grown

Blood Cells

Neural Cells

Muscle Cells

Source: BBC News.

last until the body made new white blood cells with the same defect. To counter this inevitability, they planned another treatment to re-educate the new cells so they would not attack insulin-making tissues in the pancreas. Once the diseased cells were out of the way, however, adult stem cells took over and grew new islets in 40 days.

Diabetes Reversed in the Lab

"At first we thought we had failed," Faustman recalls. She and her colleagues planned to follow up by transplanting healthy islet cells grown in their laboratory. "But the biological indicators we saw were not what we wanted for such transplants. Then we gradually realized that there were now islet cells where none had existed 40 days before. It was astonishing! We had reversed the disease without the need for transplants."

"These results are remarkable and surprising," comments David M. Nathan, the Harvard professor of medicine who will attempt to do the same experiments with humans at Massachusetts General Hospital. "We need careful studies to find out if we can delete the offending blood cells in humans in the same way that it was done in mice. Adult stem cells in these mice were apparently inactive or suppressed until cells that attacked the pancreas were removed. We don't know yet if human adult stem cells can accomplish the same regeneration. If they can, and it will take years to find out, that opens the way to treating other autoimmune diseases like multiple sclerosis and rheumatoid arthritis."

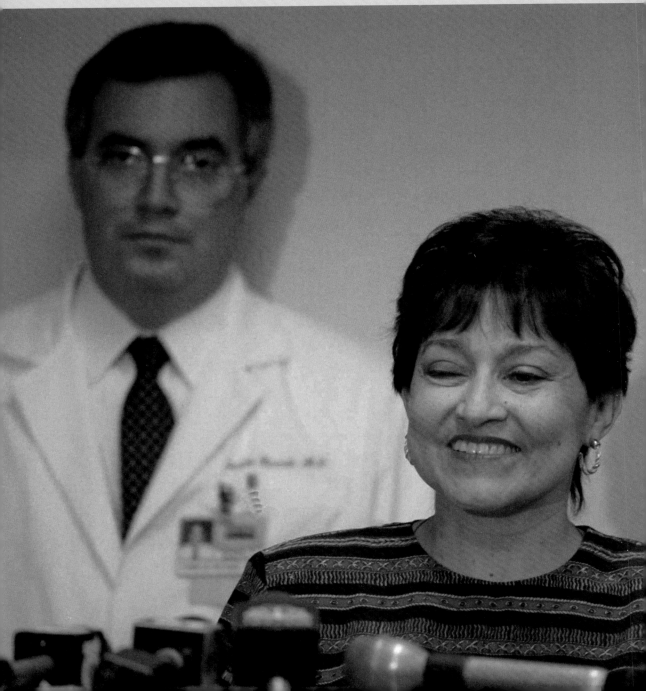

CHAPTER **3**

Personsal Perspectives on Diabetes

Della Reese Tells Her Diabetes Story

Marcia Levine Mazur

Entertainer Della Reese has had a remarkable life. In an interview with author Marcia Levine Mazur, Reese talks about her career as a gospel singer and entertainer. Mazur writes that when Reese fainted and fell down a flight of stairs while working on the set of a television show she found out that it was caused by diabetes. Della Reese shares the changes she has made after her diagnosis. They include healthier eating and exercising.

I t's a long tough road that stretches from the choir of the Church of Our Faith in Detroit, Michigan to the pinnacle of America's entertainment world. But Della Reese, one of America's best-loved celebrities, traveled it. She took the first step one steamy summer day when she was only 13. On that day the queen of gospel, Mahalia

Photo on previous page. Marta Herrera, a type 1 diabetes patient, speaks at a press conference about the reversal of her diabetes after a series of transplants. **(AP Images.)**

SOURCE: Marcia Levine Mazur, "Della Reese: 'Diabetes Will Not Make Me a Victim,'" *Diabetes Forecast*, vol. 57, July 2004, pp. 56–60. Copyright © 2004 American Diabetes Association. Reproduced by permission.

Jackson, visited her church. In need of a backup singer, Jackson heard Reese's powerful voice and signed her on the spot.

"Mahalia taught me many things, like how to sing from deep inside yourself," Reese recalls. Years later, Reese would learn a far sadder lesson from her mentor, a lesson about the devastation of untreated diabetes; Jackson died from complications of the disease.

Deloreese Patricia Early—later trimmed to Della Reese—left home when her mother died suddenly and her father remarried. She had 17 years on the calendar, 13 cents in her pocket, and a thousand reasons to make it.

Reese took almost any available job, from driving a produce track to operating a switchboard. "Some days I had to stretch one meal to cover three. But I had wonderful friends—I call them my angels—who always showed up to help me," Reese says.

Reese's Growing Career

In her early 20s, the gnawing need for money forced the singer to switch from her beloved gospel to secular music. "When you sing gospel in church, they pass a collection basket. But when you sing secular in a nightclub they pay fifty dollars a seat," she explains. (Today, Reese is known for her ability to sing gospel, pop, swing, jazz, and the blues.)

At first, Reese's unique voice and humorous onstage banter brought brief engagements in small clubs. But she was soon headlining in larger and better venues. And when she took on New York, she wowed even those tough audiences. Along the way, hit recordings ("There Will Never Be Another You," "In the Still of the Night," "Don't You Know") launched her onto the national scene.

Now it was "Miss Della Reese" appearing on top TV programs like *The Jackie Gleason Show* and *The Tonight Show*, Ed Sullivan booked her 18 times in one year; she starred at Las Vegas' posh Flamingo Hotel for nine years.

Later, she brought gospel to Vegas. "That's where they needed it," she says. "And audiences couldn't get enough of it."

(Reese reminisces about those early Vegas days. "It was a small intimate town back then and just about everyone was there: Sinatra, Sammy Davis, Dean Martin, Count Basie, Woody Herman, Harry James. It was just great.") When TV producers saw that Reese could act as well as sing, they signed her for guest appearances on hits such as *The Mod Squad*, and *Chico and the Man*.

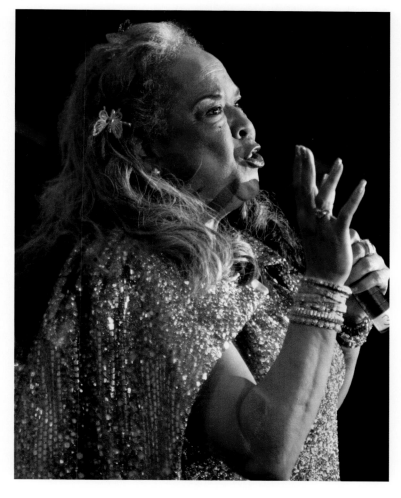

Della Reese sings in Detroit, Michigan. Overcoming obstacles and breaking down barriers have been Reese's personal and professional goals for many years. **(AP Images.)**

Quiz shows loved her, too; she became a regular on *Hollywood Squares*. Della Reese was the first black woman to host her own TV talk show. Then there were the movies. Audiences who still manage to see *Harlem Nights* howl at the fight she and Eddie Murphy have in the film.

Recognition brought gold records, Grammy, Emmy as well as Golden Globe nominations, and three NAACP Image Awards. Della Reese also has her own star on the Hollywood Walk of Fame. But don't imagine that Reese's life has been one long, happy trip to fame and stardom. Along the way there was an abusive husband, searing personal losses, and major illnesses. "Still, you'll never hear me complain about my life," Reese says.

Reese Contracted Type 2 Diabetes

Today, at age 72, Reese is probably best known as the angel Tess in CBS' long running program, *Touched by an Angel*. It was at a rehearsal for *Angel* that Reese felt faint, lost her footing, and fell down a flight of stairs. Later she developed a ferocious headache. Doctors diagnosed type 2 diabetes; Reese was stunned. "The only thing I knew about diabetes was that Ella Fitzgerald had amputations because of it, and that both she and Mahalia Jackson and other show biz friends died from its complications. I was confused and scared, but I was determined not to let any of that happen to me," Reese says.

Della Reese and her husband of over 20 years, producer/agent Franklin Thomas Lett ("I walked down the aisle with two other men, but this is my only real marriage," she explains), talked to the doctor and read all they could about diabetes. "I didn't know much about diabetes back then, but I knew one thing for sure: Ignorance and fear will kill you quicker than any disease."

Today, Reese eats healthy foods including fruits and vegetables, checks her blood glucose in the mornings and before and after meals, and takes medication daily. She also checks her blood pressure several times a week and keeps track of her cholesterol.

"I was never aware of my body before. Now I am conscious of it 24 hours a day. My body took care of me all my life, now I am going to take care of it," she adds. Although Reese still loves entertaining, she is even more passionate about her role as an ordained minister. On Sundays, you can find Reverend Della Reese-Lett conducting services at the Los Angeles church she founded some 20 years ago.

Taking Control of Her Life

Della Reese has a clear vision of how she wants her future to play out. "I don't intend to rust," she says. "I want to keep working and stay healthy as long as I can. Then one day I want to come home so tired that I just lay down in my bed and wake up with my Savior."

"You don't have to be a victim just because you have diabetes. But you do have to do whatever it takes to make changes," Della Reese explains. "For instance, I know I have to exercise, but I just hate the 'e' word —exercise. So I changed it to the 'a' word— activity. I can deal with activity."

Reese's "activities" include walking on a treadmill and riding a stationary bike. "I used to be the best friend a parking attendant ever had. Now I park a block away and walk. Sure, it's not 20 miles, but it's more than I ever walked before," she says.

> **FAST FACT**
>
> African Americans are twice as likely to develop diabetes as Caucasians. One out of seven African Americans has diabetes.

Then there's food. "Anyone with an ounce of sense knows that chickens were made to be fried in deep fat. But I found out that you can bake and broil chicken and it tastes just fine. So I had to change my mind about chicken," she explains.

For Reese, ice cream posed a real challenge. "I worked hard all my life so I could lay around and eat butter pecan ice cream in bed. But I don't do that anymore because of my diabetes. "Does that mean I can never have butter pecan ice cream again? Or sweets, for that matter? Of course not. I just can't go crazy with them. Like any changes, you have to adjust to them. But that puts you in charge, not your diabetes."

A Cruise Director Shares Her Experience with Diabetes

Cathie Goodman

In this selection Cathie Goodman, a lifelong diabetic, shares her experience as an assistant cruise director on a luxury cruise ship. She describes the thrill of receiving her job offer and the extra preparation required in planning for four months at sea. In the context of her experiences on the cruise, Goodman points out some important lessons for people with diabetes as well as others. She discusses the importance of sharing information with others. She deals with the sacrifices she has had to make and the ways she copes with events when they do not go quite right. Most important, Goodman says that diabetes should not get in the way of anyone pursuing his or her dream.

"The Mediterranean, the Black Sea, and the Amazon River? Yes, I am definitely interested," I say into the phone, barely able to conceal my excitement. "I'll call you back within the hour to confirm

SOURCE: Cathie Goodman, "Cruising with Type 1 Diabetes: Lessons from My Life at Sea," *Juvenile Diabetes Research Foundation*, July 25, 2006. www.jdrf.org. Reproduced by permission.

that everything is set." It's 4:00 on a Friday afternoon and I am shaking with adrenaline as I hang up the phone and dial my pharmacist to place an order for four months' worth of insulin. "I'll need to pick it up tomorrow," I tell him, as I scribble down the time that the pharmacy closes. I then call my insurance provider to make sure they will cover an advance on my insulin needs. I call back my recruiter at Holland America Cruise Line (HAL) and tell her I'm ready to report for duty. She replies, "That's great news! You'll arrive in Lisbon on Monday morning, where transportation is arranged to take you to the ship."

I'm thrilled. I hang up and call my parents to tell them that I was offered the job as an assistant cruise director, and that I'll be flying to Europe in 40 hours to begin my first contract! When I get to my ship, the *MS Prinsendam*, I discover that life on board is no less hectic than the day and a half I had to prepare for it. I spend the first day checking in at the human resources office, picking up my uniform, delivering my medical forms to the infirmary and befriending the nurse on duty (a wise move for someone with type 1 diabetes or juvenile diabetes). I take a tour of the ship and attend an environmental and safety orientation before I can finally freshen up with a quick shower and change into my uniform. I have about 10 minutes to catch my breath before welcoming the new passengers as we depart from Lisbon.

Being constantly on the go means I have to step up my type 1 diabetes management. Adjusting to life on a ship, in addition to the change in eating habits and constant activity, is both exciting and stressful, and all of this affects my sugar levels. I monitor my sugars more closely than usual, as I don't want my type 1 diabetes to cause any poor impressions on my new boss, coworkers, or the passengers on board.

FAST FACT

Diabetes is the sixth leading cause of death in the United States.

PERSPECTIVES ON DISEASES AND DISORDERS

Life Lessons

Lesson 1: Be Open About Your Type 1 Diabetes

I am open with my coworkers about my type 1 diabetes, and they are very supportive in response. I want them to know what to expect and how to react in case my sugars get out of whack. Sharing my juvenile diabetes has always been a good idea in my experience. People appreciate being trusted with the information and with the responsibility to take action if needed. It is also a great way to get to know my new friends. If they have experience with type 1 diabetes, we swap stories, and if not, they usually have lots of questions about the disease and how it impacts my life.

For many diabetics, managing their disease while working can be a challenge. A job aboard a cruise ship can pose special challenges for diabetics. (**AP Images.**)

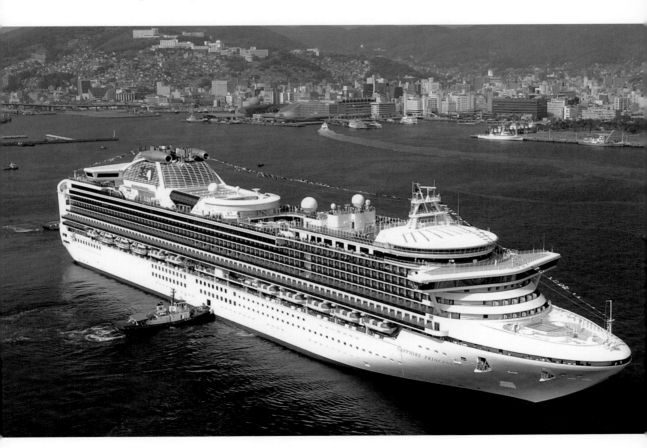

Lesson 2: There's No Such Thing as Perfect Control

After a week aboard the ship, I test my sugar before going to bed and find it at 113. All seems to be fine and I drift off to sleep. The next morning I sleep through my alarm and several phone calls from my coworker. I even manage to sleep through the cruise director pounding on my door and calling me from the hallway. He disappears for a moment and returns with the head housekeeper. As they prepare to bust into my cabin, I finally emerge from my slumber and open the door. I am groggy, but awake enough to know that I've overslept and that I'm not feeling quite right. My glucometer reads 27 and my suspicions are confirmed. I shakily devour two granola bars and a few gulps of apple juice that I have in my cabin, and get ready as quickly as I can while waiting impatiently for the glucose to have its effect.

Lesson 3: Staying Healthy Requires Some Sacrifice

Trying to fit exercise into my routine is incredibly tough when working on a cruise ship. I work long days with breaks between activities, but rarely is there enough time to fit in a good cardio workout and a shower. It is tough to stay motivated as well, as the crew gym is a dingy, cramped room at the far end of the ship. But I know I will feel better if I make the effort, so I do. I like running on the treadmill best, but I often end up doing it at midnight if I can't squeeze it in before dinner. Either way, the exercise always impacts my sugar levels, so I have to plan ahead the best I can to adjust my insulin and snacks appropriately.

Lesson 4: Always Be Prepared

Traveling the world is the best perk of the job. I have a mental checklist anytime I leave the ship—identification, money, camera, and the type 1 diabetes stuff: glucometer, snacks, and enough insulin to get me through in case something comes up and I am unable to make it back in time to sail. The ship will leave anyone behind except for the captain and the senior officers. Fortunately, there is always a port agent available to help make arrangements for any passenger or crew member left behind to catch the ship at the next port.

Lesson 5: Juvenile Diabetes Doesn't Have to Stop You from Pursuing Your Dreams

Anyone who has had to live with type 1 diabetes can tell you that it's a challenge. Although it is not something that we choose, it becomes a piece of our lives that impacts who we are. The key is not to allow it to dictate who we are. If anything, type 1 diabetes has made me determined to live my life by my terms. I love to prove to myself that I can adapt to whatever surprises life throws at me. That's one of the reasons I accepted the job with Holland America. Adjusting to life on a cruise ship certainly provided a lot of challenges. What can I say? I love a good challenge.

Mr. Universe Shares His Experience with Diabetes

Linda Von Wartburg

In the following article Linda Von Wartburg tells the amazing story of how an eleven-year-old diabetic boy became Mr. Universe. Von Wartburg explains how Doug Burns began a weight-lifting program against the advice of his doctor. She describes the challenges Doug overcame building his own gym equipment from junkyard parts. The body builder, she says, has no complications but still has to deal with diabetes. With a strict regimen of exercise and diet Doug Burns demonstrates that diabetes is not an obstacle to making dreams come true.

These days, Doug Burns is a modern Samson. The reigning Mr. Universe, he's two hundred pounds of sheer muscle and the picture of good health. Of the skinny little boy with type 1 who used to work out in the woods alone, all that remains are a wry sense of humor and an attractively self-deprecating manner. They're unexpected in a man who's triumphed in the uber-masculine world of bodybuilding, but there's a lot that's unexpected about Doug Burns.

Doug was born in Washington DC, into a family without a bit of type 1 history. His dad, who worked with NASA, moved the family to the backwoods of Mississippi when Doug was about eleven. By that time he'd had type 1 for four years, ever since a severe episode of keto-acidosis at age seven. He was what used to be called a "brittle diabetic," taking multiple injections of NPH and Regular, and he had problems with the delayed effect of the Regular. On top of that, he was trying to handle his testing with urinalysis, which could be six hours off the mark. Consequently, he was frequently in keto-acidosis or insulin shock, with constant episodes of both extreme highs and extreme lows.

As a result of his sugar management problems, Doug weighed only 58 pounds by the time he was eleven. Known as "the bag of bones," he was beaten up by pretty much everybody in school. He still remembers a girl in fifth grade who whacked him with her purse and "beat the hell out of me right in front of the class." In Mississippi he wasn't bullied as much, but as an emaciated kid with a disease no one had heard of, he was ostracized as an oddity.

At the age of twelve, in 1977, Doug came across a picture of the Biblical Samson holding a lion in a headlock. He'd never seen anything like Samson's hugely muscular body, and for the skinny, lonely boy, the sight was a revelation. That night he prayed zealously for a half hour to be changed into a Samson. When he woke the next morning as skinny as ever, he gave up on miraculous intervention and decided to take matters into his own hands.

Doug Overcame More Odds than Diabetes

Doug's physician tried to forbid him to lift weights, but he was so hell-bent on becoming Samsonesque that he ignored the doctor. Unfazed by the absence of gyms in backwoods Mississippi, he made late night forays to the junkyard and jerry-rigged his own gym with old pulleys and bags of concrete. Using an outdated issue of *Ironman* magazine as his guide, he trained in his makeshift gym in the woods come hell or high water, in the company of raccoons and bobcats, and once right through a tornado.

About the same time that he started working out, Doug got hold of a home glucose meter. His control improved immediately, and once that happened, his world opened up. No longer a bag of bones, he joined the football team, became the most valuable running back, and found a group of buddies to work out with. He and his friends would go to Wolf River, dive from the trestle, and train out in the sun with weighted dumbbells. Where the river rapids flowed through a canyon, they swam upriver like salmon.

At age fifteen, after only two years with the weights, Doug began power-lifting competitively. He placed dead last in his first competition, but by the time he graduated from high school, he had set American records in drug-free power lifting in the adult open class. Following his success as a powerlifter, he began entering bodybuilding competitions. In November 2006, the boy formerly known as "the bag of bones" became Mr. Universe.

Fitness Quest

Now the perfect model of a modern Samson, Doug is 5 foot nine inches and weighs between 187 and 200 pounds. Had it not been for diabetes, he believes, he probably would not have become a body builder. He credits his career to an overwhelming drive to overcome the disease, upped by his initial desire to fit in. And then, "Once you get pissed off about something, you say the hell with it, I'm going all the way."

Doug went on the pump only last year. He was offered a pump by MiniMed long before, but he was swimming in the Pacific Ocean on a daily basis, so he turned it down.

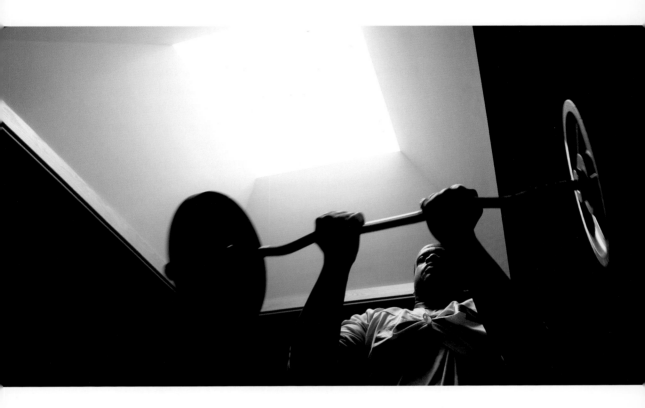

He likes his Animas pump because it's so easy to moderate his insulin doses, which change drastically depending on how he's training. When he was powerlifting, he was much heavier, in the 220s, and his cardiovascular work was next to nothing. When he began competing in bodybuilding, however, he did constant cardio, lost twenty pounds, and lowered his body fat from 14 percent to 4.7 percent. As a result, he had to come down 87 percent on his insulin, dropping from a daily 50 to 60 units of basal insulin down to eleven units a day. By the time he was ready for the show, one unit of insulin was more than enough to cover the same amount of carbs that twelve units had covered before.

When he's getting ready for a contest, Doug moves his testing frequency way, way up. Because his body fat is coming down so drastically, he starts using cardiovascular

A nutritious diet and exercise are important parts of a healthy lifestyle, and they can play a significant role in managing diabetes. (AP Images.)

work to chase his glucose. He begins pulling off of bolus injections; instead, he moderates what he's eating in conjunction with whatever training he's doing. So he takes glucose when he knows he's going to need it, and then does aerobic work right afterward to "just burn the heck out of it." As his body fat keeps dropping, the whole mechanism keeps improving and improving. . . .

Doug's never run into any prejudice against diabetes in the gym, though he is very open about testing and his pump. People sometimes give him the eye, thinking that insulin might be advantageous in competition, but insulin is of no use to him in that respect because if his insulin ever goes high, he can't shed body fat and get lean enough to compete. For competitions, he brings his insulin dosage down to probably less than that of a non-diabetic person. . . .

Doug loves ocean swimming, but does most of his cardio work in the hills of California. He also hits the elliptical pretty frequently and the treadmill on a regular basis. One of the most effective ways he's found to combine both aerobic and anaerobic exercise is with full-on sprinting. He does 40s and 100s, and he finds that it literally gives a hammering to his metabolism, so he's geared up for the next ten hours.

Fitness Training Keeps Vitals in Great Shape

Doug's last A1c [a test showing average blood sugar level] was 5.9. His blood pressure is on the verge of being too low, about 100 over 70. His resting pulse rate when he won the Southern States was 39. He tries to keep his sugar readings super tight by forcing himself to pay attention, and his current blood sugars vacillate from the high fifties to 170. He tries to stay between 70 and 110.

Doug has no complications of diabetes at all, and he attributes this mostly to his aerobic work. He has talked with scientists at length about the effect that cardio has on the buildup of AGEs (advanced glycosylated end products), and he's convinced that the increased blood flow, coupled with adequate to higher levels of water intake, acts like turpentine cleaning a dirty pipe. He believes that active cardio work over an extended period of time is unbeatable for keeping the vessels open.

Doug emphasizes that for him, it's not about diet and exercise: It's about exercise and diet. Exercise is primary. He says that diets are misleading, in that they promise that you can simply eat your way to health. He does have a particular diet that he follows, leaning a little more on protein. He "eats very, very clean" throughout the week and gives himself one day to enjoy whatever he feels like having. He loves Cajun food with a passion, and his favorite beer, Chili Creek, is spiced up by a big hot pepper inside the bottle.

Doug doesn't take any meds except children's aspirin, but he takes a lot of supplements, including isolated whey plus whey concentrate, multi-vitamins and minerals, essential fatty acids, L-glutamine and carnitine. He notes a distinct beneficial effect when he takes supplements, which he uses to advantage when preparing for competition: He works without supplements until he is in the best possible shape, and then adds the supplements to take it up a notch. He notes that his way is the antithesis of the public's inclination to take the magic potion right from the get-go. He has always done the work first and then used the supplements as an adjunct to the hard work. . . .

Doug developed his self-deprecating sense of humor as a way of disarming his childhood adversaries, and it's been part of him ever since. Poking fun at himself after a low blood sugar makes the incident easier to stomach and less daunting to others. When he makes light of something, it's a way of defining it for himself and for

> ## FAST FACT
>
> Half of all diabetics will die from heart disease and related ailments. An additional 20 percent will die from kidney failure.

everyone else too. Recently, however, during an incident which cannot be lightened with humor, he was beaten by police during an episode of hypoglycemia. Despite his medic alert jewelry and wallet cards, the police assumed that he was intoxicated. The incident serves to underscore the fact that police and security guards need to be far better educated about diabetes and hypoglycemia.

Doug says that when he speaks at diabetes conferences, the kids in the audience sometimes assume that because he's a successful professional athlete, diabetes somehow went away and doesn't apply to him anymore. He's quick to emphasize that he faces the same daily struggles that they do. He always has to pay attention, and the pitfalls never cease to exist. Kids sometimes feel that when they go low or have a bad day, they're all alone, the only ones who have such problems. When they hear that someone who's set a record still has to struggle just like they do, it's a revelation to them. Doug makes it clear that he still has bad days and doesn't feel like training, but that's where his sense of discipline comes in.

Diabetes has been a spur to Doug. He believes that the discipline required to manage the disease ultimately benefited him, carrying over into the discipline that he needed to succeed as an athlete. He advises kids to accept diabetes for what it is, simply an obstacle like any other, one that they can use instead of letting it use them. He tells kids, number one, don't think of yourself as defective merchandise because that's just not the case, and number two, pursue your dream no matter how far-fetched it might seem. Just make diabetes come along with you. Never give up.

GLOSSARY

autoimmune disease   A disease in which the body attacks its own cells. Diabetes is an autoimmune disease.

body mass index   An index used to measure a person's weight against a standard. The BMI is equal to weight in kilograms divided by height in meters, with that number divided by height in meters a second time.

carbohydrates   A source of energy typically found in grain, fruit, and vegetables. Eating carbohydrates increases blood sugar levels.

chronic   Having a long duration. Diabetes is a chronic disease.

diabetes   A chronic disease in which the body cannot use glucose for fuel because the pancreas does not produce enough insulin or the body cannot properly use the insulin that is produced, causing abnormally high levels of sugar in the blood.

dialysis   The process of cleaning the blood of impurities with a machine. People whose kidneys have failed must have dialysis several times a week to filter their blood.

endocrinologist   A physician that specializes in diseases of glands, including the pancreas.

Exubera   The first inhalable insulin.

fructose   A form of sugar found in fruits and vegetables. It is digested more slowly than glucose.

gestational diabetes   Diabetes that occurs during pregnancy. This form of diabetes usually disappears after the birth. Women who experience gestational diabetes are at a higher risk for developing type 2 diabetes later in life.

glucose	Sugar carried by the blood to cells throughout the body. It is the body's main source of energy.
hematopoietic	Pertaining to the formation of blood or blood cells; hematopoietic stem cells in bone marrow build all of the elements of the immune system.
hyperglycemia	High levels of blood sugar. Hyperglycemia is a symptom of diabetes and is treated with insulin injections. Extreme levels of hyperglycemia is called ketoacidosis.
hypoglycemia	Low levels of blood sugar caused by high insulin levels; in terms of diabetes, this condition is also referred to as an "insulin reaction."
insulin	The hormone produced by the pancreas that controls the amount of glucose that enters the cells of the body.
islet cells	The cells of the pancreas that manufacture hormones. Alpha cells produce glucagon, which can raise blood sugar. Beta cells produce insulin.
ketoacidosis	A life-threatening condition in which the blood sugar and acidity of the blood are both high. Symptoms include nausea, vomiting, rapid breathing, drowsiness, and weakness. This is a serious condition and requires a doctor's care.
ketones	Acid compounds that form in the blood when the body breaks down fats and proteins.
lethargy	A symptom of diabetes in which a person feels an abnormal drowsiness.
morbidity rate	The rate at which people develop a particular disease compared to the population at large.
mortality rate	The rate at which people die from a particular disease compared to the population at large.
nephropathy	Kidney damage, frequently as a complication from diabetes. Kidney failure makes it necessary to rely on dialysis to filter blood.

neuropathy	Nerve damage, frequently a complication of diabetes. Peripheral neuropathy is numbness in the feet and legs.
obesity	The condition of weighing more than 20 percent more than one's ideal body weight. Obesity is closely correlated with type 2 diabetes.
pancreas	The organ, located behind the stomach, that produces insulin.
retinopathy	Disease of the retina, which may be diabetes related. Retinopathy can result in blindness if not treated.
transplant	To transfer (tissue or an organ) from one body or body part to another.
type 1 diabetes	Also known as juvenile diabetes; this type of diabetes is brought on by a combination of factors, including a genetic predisposition for the disease or a virus. It typically appears between childhood and early adulthood.
type 2 diabetes	Also known as adult-onset diabetes; this type of diabetes is usually related to obesity. While traditionally thought to be an adult disease, more younger people, even children, are contracting it.

CHRONOLOGY

B.C.   circa   Demetrios of Apameia in ancient Greece first uses
            100   the word "diabetes."

A.D.   1425   The word "diabetes" is used in an English book for the
                     first time.

            1674   In England Thomas Willis observes that the urine of
                     people with diabetes is sweet. He begins a period of
                     research into diabetes in England.

            1869   Paul Langerhans, a medical student in Berlin, discovers
                     the cells in the pancreas that produce an unknown sub-
                     stance later referred to as insulin. These cells become
                     known as the Islets of Langerhans.

            1908   George Ludwig Zuelzer isolates a pancreatic substance
                     that he injects into five patients with diabetes. Their
                     blood sugar level goes down but they have side effects
                     that are not acceptable.

            1909   Jean de Meyer (Belgium) proposes the name "insulin"
                     for the unknown substance in the pancreas.

            1911   S.R. Benedict develops a technique to measure sugar in
                     urine. His formula becomes known as Benedict's Solu-
                     tion.

            1921   Frederick Banting at the University of Toronto isolates
                     insulin from the pancreas of a dog.

1922	Leonard Thompson in Toronto becomes the first human to be treated with insulin.
1923	Eli Lilly and Company begins to produce insulin on a commercial basis.
1925	The first home tests for sugar in urine become available.
1940s	A link is made between diabetes and long-term complications (kidney and eye disease).
1960	The radioimmunological assay (RIA) test is developed by Rosalyn Yalow and Solomon Berson to measure insulin. Yalow wins a Nobel Prize in 1977 for her work.
1964	The first test strips for testing blood sugar become available. A drop of blood is left on the paper for one minute and then washed off. The color left is compared to a chart to determine the level of blood sugar.
1966	University of Minnesota surgeons perform the world's first pancreas transplant.
1970	The first blood sugar meter becomes available. The use of laser therapy begins to slow or stop the onset of blindness caused by diabetic retinopathy (eye disease caused by diabetes).
1976	The glycosylated hemoglobin test (A1c) is developed and introduced.
1978	The National Diabetes Information Clearinghouse is established to provide information about the disease to the medical community and the public.

1979   Type 1 and type 2 diabetes are formally recognized by the American Diabetes Association. Type 1 is also called Insulin Dependent Diabetes Mellitus (IDDM), and type 2 is called Non-Insulin Dependent Diabetes Mellitus (NIDDM).

1990s   The introduction of external insulin pumps affords better control and makes administering insulin easier.

1993   The results of the Diabetes Control and Complications Trial are published. The trial shows that more frequent doses of insulin that are adjusted for the level of activity will delay the onset of complications such as eye, kidney, and nerve disease.

1997   The American Diabetes Association determines blood-glucose standards: a) Less than 110 mg/dL is considered normal, b) 111 to 125 mg/dL is considered to be impaired glucose tolerance, and c) 126 mg/dL or greater is considered to be diabetic.

2003   The names "IDDM" and "NIDDM" are dropped. The impaired glucose level is changed to 100 to 125 mg/dL.

2005   The Food and Drug Administration authorizes inhalable insulin.

ORGANIZATIONS TO CONTACT

The editors have compiled the following list of organizations concerned with the issues debated in this book. The descriptions are derived from materials provided by the organizations. All have publications or information available for interested readers. Most of these publications are available online and can be downloaded for free in HTML or PDF format. The list was compiled on the date of publication of the present volume; the information provided here may change. Be aware that many organizations take several weeks or longer to respond to inquiries, so allow as much time as possible.

American Diabetes Association (ADA)
1701 N. Beauregard St.
Alexandria, VA 22311
(800) 342-2383
www.diabetes.org

The American Diabetes Association is a nonprofit advocacy organization dedicated to preventing and curing diabetes. The ADA funds research, publishes information, and offers support to people with diabetes and their families. The Web site offers free e-newsletters, including *Diabetes World* and *ADA's Monthly Spotlight.*

American Dietetic Association
120 S. Riverside Plaza, Suite 2000
Chicago, IL 60606
(800) 877-1600
www.eatright.org

This association provides information about dietary research and also supplies support and information to help people with diabetes assess and modify their diet. The Web site offers access to the *Journal of the American Dietetic Association* and provides its members with newsletters, including *ADA Student Scoop* and *ADA Times.*

Canadian Diabetes Association
National Life Building
1400-522 University Ave.
Toronto ON M5G 2R5
Canada
www.diabetes.ca

The Canadian Diabetes Association provides bilingual (English and French) support for people with diabetes and their families. It lobbies all levels of government to create public awareness of diabetes as a growing public health issue. This association publishes *Beyond the Basics: Meal Planning for Healthy Eating, Diabetes Prevention and Management,* and the e-newsletter *Diabetes Current.*

Centers for Disease Control and Prevention (CDC)
1600 Clifton Rd.
Atlanta, GA 30333
(404) 639-3311
www.cdc.gov/health/
diabetes.htm

The CDC is a division of the U.S. Department of Health and Human Services and offers up-to-date information on diabetes, including research, FAQs, and activities of the CDC in finding new treatments and a cure. The CDC's Web site offers fact sheets, reports, and guides, in addition to Diabetes Public Health Resource publications, which are free of charge.

Diabetic Exercise and Sports Association (DESA)
8001 Montcastle Dr.
Nashville, TN 37221
(800) 898-4322
www.diabetes-exercise.org

Athletics pose challenges to those with diabetes. This organization shares information on what types of exercise are appropriate and what are not, as well as diet and nutrition information. Members of its Web site are also offered access to the DESA newsletter.

International Diabetes Center (IDC)
3800 Park Nicollet Blvd.
St. Louis Park, MN 55416-2699
(952) 993-3393
www.parknicollet.com/diabetes

Part of the Park Nicollet Clinic, the International Diabetes Center offers education classes for people with diabetes and training programs for health professionals. IDC also provides treatment services in adult and pediatric clinics in addition to supporting and conducting diabetes research. The organization publishes nutrition guides for patients, low-literacy patient education booklets, a curriculum for health professionals, and general publications related to diabetes, including their *Fast Food Facts* book.

Joslin Diabetes Center
One Joslin Pl.
Boston, MA 02215
(617) 732-2400

The Joslin Clinic supports diabetes research and provides medical care for people with diabetes. The Joslin Diabetes Center provides general information and literature about diabetes, including the Joslin Library of diabetes data.

Juvenile Diabetes Research Foundation (JDRF)
120 Wall St.
New York, NY 10005
(800) 533-CURE (2873)
www.jdrf.org

The JDRF supports research directed at finding a cure for type 1 diabetes. The JDRF provides information for people who are newly diagnosed with diabetes as well as an online support team to provide practical help. The JDRF publishes magazines including *Countdown* and *Countdown for Kids,* and e-newsletters including *Emerging Technologies in Diabetes Research* and *Life with Diabetes.*

National Diabetes Information Clearinghouse
One Information Way
Bethesda, MD 20892
(800) 860-8747
www.diabetes.niddk.nih.gov

This clearinghouse provides information about diabetes to people with diabetes, their families, doctors, and other health care professionals. The Web site also offers free, easy-to-read publications in both English and Spanish.

National Eye Institute (NEI)—National Eye Health Education Program
Box 20/20
Bethesda, MD 20892
(301) 496-5248
(800) 869-2020
www.nei.nih.gov

NEI—part of the National Institutes of Health—supports research to develop effective treatments for diabetic eye disease. The institute's National Eye Health Education Program promotes public and professional awareness of the importance of early diagnosis and treatment of diabetic eye disease. The NEI publishes the newsletter *Outlook Information Bulletin,* as well as brochures, fact sheets, and reports.

National Institute of Diabetes and Digestive and Kidney Disease (NIDDK)
31 Center Dr.
USC2560, Bldg. 31,
Room 9A-04
Bethesda, MD 20892
(301) 496-3683
www2.niddk.nih.gov

The NIDDK is a part of the National Institutes of Health, a government organization that tracks progress being made in the treatment of diabetes and digestive and kidney diseases. It also conducts and supports research into these diseases. NIDDK offers statistics and a selection of publications about these diseases.

FOR FURTHER READING

Books

American Diabetes Association, *American Diabetes Association Complete Guide to Diabetes.* New York: Bantam, 2006.

Neal Barnard and Bryanna Clark Grogan, *Dr. Neal Barnard's Program for Reversing Diabetes.* New York: Rodale, 2007.

Gretchen Beaker, *The First Year: Type 2 Diabetes.* New York: Marlowe, 2001.

Jennie Brand-Miller, Kaye Foster-Powell, Stephen Colagiuri, and Alan Barclay, *The New Glucose Revolution for Diabetes.* New York: Marlowe, 2007.

Maria Collazo-Clavell, *Mayo Clinic Guide on Managing Diabetes.* Rochester, MN: Mayo Clinic, 2006.

Francine R. Kaufman, *Diabesity: The Obesity-Diabetes Epidemic That Threatens America—and What We Must Do to Stop It.* New York: Bantam, 2005.

Andrew J. Krentz, *Emergencies in Diabetes: Diagnosis, Management, and Prevention.* New York: Wiley, 2004.

Boyd E. Metzger, *American Medical Association Guide to Living with Diabetes.* New York: Wiley, 2006.

David M. Nathan, *Beating Diabetes.* Cambridge, MA: Harvard University Press, 2005.

Alan L. Rubin, *Diabetes for Dummies.* 2nd ed. New York: Wiley, 2004.

Periodicals

Jerry Adler and Claudia Kolb, "Diabetes: It Strikes 16 Million Americans. Are You at Risk?" *Newsweek*, September 4, 2000.

William E. Cayley Jr., "The Role of Exercise in Patients with Type 2 Diabetes," *American Family Physician*, February 1, 2007.

Nancy Clark, "Sinister Sweets and Toxic Treats," *American Fitness*, January/February 2007.

Ruth Colagiuri, Stephen Colugiuri, Derek Yach, and Stig Pramming, "The Answer to Diabetes Prevention: Science, Surgery, Service Delivery, or Social Policy?" *American Journal of Public Health*, September 2006.

Countdown, "Diabetes Research and the Scientific Process," Winter 2007.

Economist, "An American Epidemic," February 17, 2007.

Yvette Getch, Foram Bhukhanwala, and Stacey Neuharth-Prichett, "Strategies for Helping Children with Diabetes in Elementary and Middle Schools," *Teaching Exceptional Children*, January/February 2007.

Harvard Heart Letter, "Blood Pressure Drugs Can Boost Blood Sugar," February 2007.

Manon Khazrai, "Developing Food Strategies for the Prevention of Diabetes," *Functional Foods & Nutraceuticals*, December 2006.

Kathie Lipinski, "Living with Diabetes the Reiki Way," *Reiki News Magazine*, Spring 2007.

Peter Pompei, "Diabetes Mellitus in Later Life," *Generations*, Fall 2006.

Susan V. Ponchilla, "Diabetes Management and Visual Impairment," *Journal of Visual Impairment and Blindness*, special supplement, 2006.

Pulse, "Can Diet and Exercise Prevent Diabetes?" February 15, 2007.

Robert E. Rakel, "The Role of the Family Physician in the Diagnosis and Treatment of Type 2 Diabetes Mellitus," *Journal of the Family Physician*, December 2006.

Ron Ramsing and Eddie Hill, "How Camps Can Help Adolescents Self-Manage Diabetes," *Camping Magazine*, January/February 2007.

Kate Ruder, "Diabetes During Pregnancy Carries a Lifelong Risk of Type 2 for Mother and Child," *Diabetes Forecast*, December 2006.

Saturday Evening Post, "Diabetes: Don't Forget the Fiber," July/August 2006.

Douglas Scott, "Dealing with Diabetes," *Current Health*, September 2006.

Vera Tweed, "How to Put the Brakes on Diabetes," *Better Nutrition*, November 2006.

Mary Annette Wright and Susan J. Appel, "Inhaled Insulin: Breathing New Life into Diabetes Therapy," *Nursing*, January 2007.

INDEX